COMBINING
FOR LIFE

FOOD COMBINING FOR LIFE

The Health Success of the Century

DORIS GRANT

Thorsons
An Imprint of HarperCollinsPublishers

Thorsons
An Imprint of HarperCollins*Publishers*
77-85 Fulham Palace Road,
Hammersmith, London W6 8JB

1160 Battery Street,
San Francisco, California 94111–1213

Published by Thorsons 1995
1 3 5 7 9 10 8 6 4 2

A catalogue record for this book
is available from the British Library

ISBN 0 7225 3165 6

Printed in Great Britain by
HarperCollinsManufacturing Glasgow

This book is lovingly dedicated to
Gordon
my highly supportive and helpful
93-years-young husband.

Contents

Acknowledgements

❧

I would like to express my gratitude to the following people for help and assistance so willingly given me while preparing this book:

Dr Walter Yellowlees, for providing me with valuable references and quotations, and for carefully guiding my footsteps over many pitfalls while traversing the nutritional wilderness; Dr Kenneth Vickery, for his constant, splendid encouragement and helpful suggestions, and especially for overcoming his original fear that in promoting the Hay System over the years I was nutritionally 'going off course down a side alley'; Dr Hans Moolenburgh, for his frequent helpful letters and suggestions, and encouraging interest in the unfolding of this book; my daughter, Dr Elizabeth Stanley, for constructive and welcome criticisms; and Eileen Brooksbank, for valuable eleventh-hour help with a difficult chapter.

I particularly want to thank Jean Joice for her splendid foreword and for being, as always, such a tower of strength, especially when problems arose over the book's construction; Barbara Lewis, for virtually faultless typing and her helpful appreciation and assessment of each chapter as it took shape; Nora Wingate, for drawing my attention to Dr G. Orth of Leutkirch, Germany, and his apt vindication of Hay principles described in Chapter 4; Leslie Moule, for so opportunely providing a piece of important information for Chapter 6; 'The Thorsons Team' for all their splendid help and encouragement; and, last, to food combiners worldwide whose grateful and enthusiastic letters have made my daily postbag so enthralling for so many years.

Foreword

One of my most vivid memories is of the lady from Suffolk who rushed up to me at a book-signing exclaiming, 'Look at my hands!' I looked, but could see nothing unusual, and said so. 'That's the whole point,' she replied. 'They are back to normal now, but three months ago they were so swollen and crippled with arthritis that I could hardly use them. The pain was dreadful and I was afraid that I would never be able to do any fine needlework again.' She was so thrilled with the marvellous improvement in her hands and general health after discovering the Hay System that she had made the journey to Norwich to tell me about it and have her copy of *Food Combining for Health* signed by one of the authors.

This kind of experience is the greatest reward that any health writer can have and, as Doris Grant recounts in this, her latest and most inspiring book, one that has come her way many times over her long career. Although Doris resolutely refuses to claim any credit for the wonderful results that follow from the way of eating originally pioneered by Dr William Howard Hay, it is nevertheless true that her enthusiastic championship of sound nutrition must have helped countless families to better health over the years.

My own family was a case in point. My mother came across an article by Doris in *Housewife* many years ago and decided to try her hand at the Grant Loaf. She never looked back, and the delicious, nutty, wholewheat loaf literally became 'our daily bread'. We children soon became zealous bakers too, a habit which has persisted to this day. I have never willingly eaten white bread since, and it is entirely due to Doris that we discovered the benefits of fibre (then known as 'roughage') in our food long before Doctors Cleave and Burkitt convinced the medical establishment of its value.

Yet more health benefits were to follow. My father, browsing in his favourite bookshop one day, noticed a book called *Dear Housewives* by Doris Grant which he promptly bought and gave to my mother. So persuasive was the author that the Grant Loaf habit was swiftly followed by the salad habit and the less-sugar habit (not so easy to acquire!). We were also discouraged from eating processed foods and, alas, chips (we rather regretted the loss of my mother's delicious deep-fried chips!).

So it was that I grew up with Doris Grant principles, as it were, firmly instilled, and there must be thousands of households that have been persuaded to follow a healthy, wholefood lifestyle by the enthusiasm and sheer energy that have radiated from the pages of Doris's many books and articles over the years. In due course I made 'the loaf' for my own children and also discovered, quite by chance, an earlier 'Doris' book of

menus for the Hay System. As I was finding it difficult
to shed the surplus pounds acquired during my second
pregnancy, I put this unfamiliar regime to the test.
Needless to say, the extra weight soon disappeared.

It was not until the publication of *Your Daily Food*,
however, that Doris and I actually met. At this time I
was working for Anglia Television and seized the
opportunity to interview Doris about her latest book.
We made a short film for Anglia's afternoon
programme 'About Women', in which Doris demonstrated her famous loaf.

This first meeting took place over 20 years ago, and
since then we have enjoyed a productive working part-
nership and a warm and enduring friendship. No-one
could fail to be inspired by Doris's total dedication to
the cause of better nutrition based on sound, common-
sense principles, and there can be few writers who
have done more to improve the nation's health.

It was the impression made by her own youthful
looks and amazing energy coupled with an equally
astonishing capacity for both sheer hard work and
enjoyment of life that caused me to take another look at
the Hay way of eating. Although I had no specific
health problem to overcome, I was sufficiently
convinced by my improved stamina and wellbeing to
jump at the opportunity to work with Doris on *Food
Combining for Health*.

Since then, the evidence of the success of the Hay
System in resolving health problems, both physical
and mental, has accumulated to such an extent that
Doris has once more taken up her pen, and we must
rejoice that she has.

Always a prophet ahead of her time, Doris Grant

has written another inspiring book, a celebration of her outstanding contribution to our knowledge of nutrition; and the fact that it is published in the year of her 90th birthday will give hope and encouragement to all who read it. To the young it offers the possibility of buoyant health and happiness; to older readers the realization that life can be fun and full of promise at any age. In Doris's own words, 'we can all be as well as we wish to be', and this remarkable book, the distillation of a lifetime's experience of food combining, will show you how.

Jean Joice

Introduction

After the remarkable success of *Food Combining for Health*, written over 10 years ago with my splendid co-author Jean Joice, and with due regard to the close proximity of my nineties, I decided it was high time to put my feet up. And so, with great determination, I decided: *no more books*!

This decision, alas, was gradually undermined during the past few years by a number of important matters which were daily assuming more urgency.

First (and most important of all), there was in my study an enormous and ever-increasing collection of letters from very grateful readers. They contained such astonishing accounts of benefits experienced on adopting the Hay System that, somehow or other, a fair sample of them had to be recorded before the letters landed one day in the local incinerator! This has now been done, and I hope you will find the letters in Chapters 3 and 4 not only compulsive and inspiring reading but also powerful vindication of Dr Hay's food combining principles.

Second, the degenerative diseases are on the increase, in both adults and children, despite an array of expensive modern drugs and new vaccines for this and that disease. The Hay System costs nothing, can do no harm, and appears to deal effectively, and often quickly, with many if not most of today's degenerative ailments. Its undoubted success, as detailed in the chapters mentioned above, now urgently calls for careful research. As Dr Walter Yellowlees points out in Chapter 7: 'If the healing power of food combining was confirmed and achieved wide acceptance in the NHS, the relief of suffering and saving of wealth would be incalculable.'

Third, research for my books during the past 50 years or more has convinced me beyond doubt of one vitally important truth – that the *primary* cause of most disease is not the outside germ or virus, but the inside state of the body – the 'terrain' – created by the way we eat and live. The implication of this is of great importance, as Dr Hay and many other nutritionally enlightened physicians in modern times have been consistently pointing out: germs and viruses are only effective if faulty nutrition, continuing for years, has prepared the 'terrain' by breaking down the body's remarkable inbuilt defence mechanisms. This is the theme throughout this book.

Last, the medical sceptics are still refuting Dr Hay's starch/protein principle, despite the ease with which it can be tested in a matter of days or weeks on a chronically rebellious digestion. I am, nevertheless, deeply grateful to these 'apostles of orthodoxy', for without their determined dismissal of the Hay System as a 'load of rubbish', this book would never have been written!

In it you will read astonishing evidence that food

combining really works. If you are already a convert, you will feel vindicated. If you have heard about food combining and are not sure if it works, here is the proof. If you have been suffering from chronic ill health, you may feel prompted to try it for yourself. And, if you are an out-and-out sceptic, I hope that you will be persuaded by the words of ordinary people that you can give a remarkable boost to your health by eating the Hay way. It is still not known exactly how it works, but the overwhelming evidence suggests that it does – for life.

1

My Personal Experience

One of my most vivid recollections is, at the age of nine, feasting on a forbidden but deliciously outsized chocolate Easter egg. Alas, my transgression was quickly followed by severe stomach pains which landed me on the operating table of the local hospital where my appendix was promptly removed.

From then onwards, throughout my school-days at Banff Academy, I experienced bouts of nagging indigestion. When my school-days were over, I started a five-year diploma course at the famous Glasgow School of Art. During these years, whilst living in a student hostel, my long-suffering stomach was daily subjected to the indigestible mixtures of orthodox institutional catering – it soon went on strike! I can well remember, after some particularly indigestible meals, rushing up to my room to roll on my bed in the hope of easing the pain. I can also clearly remember the frequent colds and constant tiredness which I experienced during those years of hostel living.

At the end of five years I had gained a diploma and post-diploma, and won the art school's top prize – the 'Prix de Rome'. As I was engaged to be married, however, I (rightly) had to renounce this coveted prize in favour of the student with the next highest marks to mine who, unlike me, intended making art his career.

During my early married life the nagging indigestion and tiredness continued, but with home cooking they were much less severe. In my late 20s, however, disaster struck – while sipping a very sweet sugary cocktail at a party, my limbs suddenly seized up, *I couldn't move*, and I had to be carried around for the rest of the evening. Next day, my doctor diagnosed rheumatoid trouble in my joints and prescribed the usual medicine. This had no effect whatsoever; I got steadily worse and was reduced to climbing stairs on my hands and knees. It was then that a doctor-cousin came to the rescue with a most unorthodox medical prescription. It consisted of three columns of foods – proteins, starches and acid fruits – with the instruction: 'Don't mix foods that fight!'

Within a week, indigestion of 15 years' duration was resolved.

Within two weeks, I lost four pounds of excess weight – an unexpected bonus – and developed an ability to think more clearly than formerly. I also experienced a great general feeling of well-being.

Within four weeks, all the rheumatoid pains had gone and have never returned. From that day I never looked back.

By the end of the year I felt a new woman — tireless, filled with a new energy never before experienced. The more difficult the task, the more I enjoyed it as a challenge to my new-found health and abilities.

Yet, apart from not eating meat or acid fruits

(apples, oranges, pears, grapefruit, etc.) with bread or sugared foods, I was still eating the usual everyday foods – including white bread and sugar and all the refined, processed foods which are now taboo in a healthy diet. That it worked despite this tends to discredit the frequent argument put forward today by 'sceptics' that any benefit experienced from eating the food combining way is entirely because of a change over to wholefoods

I had been almost a year on my new diet when I discovered and studied Dr William Howard Hay's inspiring book *A New Health Era*, and found that there was much more to the Hay way of eating than 'not mixing foods that fight'! As a result, my diet and health improved still further, and I came to the remarkable conclusion that I could be as well as I wished to be; that, in fact, *we hold our health in our own hands to a very large extent.*

During 64 years of eating the Hay way, I was to prove this truth up to the hilt. My health has been remarkable: I have had no illnesses or allergies; for the past 30 years I have had none of the usual bouts of 'flu or frequent colds – encouraging evidence of the improved efficiency of my immune system – and no arthritic pains. And, I have experienced none of the usual female miseries – cellulite; unmanageable lank hair that requires washing every few days; PMT and painful periods – and I sailed happily through 'the change'.

Moreover, I have not had the slightest need for weight-watching; my weight keeps a steady normal for my height (just under 7 stones for my 5 ft.), and I still have the slim figure of my 20s. My energy, too, seems inexhaustible. While writing this book I worked most evenings till 11 o'clock or midnight without feeling tired and was still quite ready to get up at 6.15 a.m. and prepare breakfast for two at 6.40 a.m. Fortunately, I fall asleep quickly and sleep soundly!

During the past 30 years, however, I have had recurring bouts of severe pain from adhesions, *which had nothing to do with the state of my health* but were the painful legacy from a badly done Caesarian at the birth of my first child. These adhesions necessitated four operations and five hospitalizations for what is called 'conservative' treatment. Thanks to my excellent health, the remarkable speed of my recoveries from these operations astonished both doctors and surgeons. At a check-up a few weeks after one of these operations I well remember my surgeon remarking: 'Mrs Grant, you have had some shockingly-badly-done surgery and had it not been for your lifestyle you might have been pushing up the daisies a long time ago!'

The Caesarian was indeed so badly done that it was necessary to operate again a year later to remove or mitigate its disastrous effects. These were such that the doctor and surgeon had to warn me that I would never be able to have another child. They reckoned, however, without the wonderful healing powers of the body when aided with compatible eating. Nine years after the birth of my first child I produced with ease a much-longed-for second child. This second birth, according to my gynaecologist, was 'a textbook demonstration of a beautifully normal birth'.

It must, nevertheless, be admitted that departing from orthodox eating habits was not an easy path to begin with. Relatives and friends, especially medical friends, pooh-pooh'd the idea of a connection between food and health! Most of them regarded me as a crank and thought I had taken leave of my senses, whereas, in fact, I was just beginning to come to them! Friends argued that I was going to miss out on all the joys of eating: 'What, no sugar in your tea? – no sugary desserts? – no biscuits and cheese? – no apple tart? You poor thing!'

I was astonished, however, to find that food is much more enjoyable when of the right kind – fresh, whole, unprocessed and *properly combined* (and I *could* now and then bend the rules and have my favourite dessert, thus having the best of both worlds). I was even more astonished to find that my new diet was no diet whatsoever, nor was it a diet to follow for a short time as a temporary cure for a specific condition, or to lose weight. Rather it was a philosophy of living – *a lifestyle* – involving a return to properly constituted foods and common-sense principles which ensure health and fitness and greatly minimize the necessity for medical treatment. The fear, also, of ill-health in advancing years is largely removed.

Little did I know in those early days that the healthy policies I had adopted – thought by so many people at that time as 'cranky' and 'way out' – would be very widely accepted by the end of the 1980s, and hailed as eminently sensible and desirable into the 1990s. Little did I know, also, that in the early 1980s I was to write, with Jean Joice, a book called *Food Combining for Health*, and that its phenomenal success and enthusiastic reception world-wide was to reveal how desperately it was needed.

By 1936, weekly articles on The Hay System appeared in a well-known national Sunday newspaper – the now defunct *Sunday Graphic*. The articles, however, were badly written and, Hay-wise, full of errors. I kept on saying so to my husband until, in exasperation, he shouted: 'For goodness sake, woman, ring the *Graphic* editor and tell him exactly what you think of the articles.' I did so. The editor evidently decided that I sounded as if I knew what I was talking about, and promptly asked me to visit him in his London office. There, two editors welcomed me with obvious relief; they had been receiving continual complaints about the number of errors in the articles. Would I take on the job of writing them? When I demurred, pointing out that I had done no journalism, the reply was: 'No matter, we will send a journalist to your home in Hertfordshire every week. All you will have to do is talk to him and he will put the article together.'

For the first article this was fine. Then my Scots independence asserted itself: 'I'm jolly well going to write my own articles!' And so I wrote the second article, thoroughly enjoyed doing so, and posted it to the *Graphic* office. To my astonishment, the Editor-in-Chief telephoned me himself as soon as he had read it: 'Mrs Grant, you are showing signs of being a born journalist – we are publishing your article word for word.' From then onwards I wrote a weekly full-page article, and very soon the *Graphic* appended my name to it.

These articles continued for over nine months and generated enormous interest, bringing into the *Graphic* office 300 to 500 letters every week. The

Graphic, moreover, gave the articles much publicity, even advertising them on the sides of London buses, to the great excitement of family and friends.

The letters from *Graphic* readers were an education and most revealing; their almost monotonous burden was the virtual failure of medical treatment *where the degenerative diseases of civilization are concerned*. The 'cure', in fact, was frequently described as being worse than the disease.

As the weeks passed, however, enthusiastic converts began sending in many accounts of remarkable benefits from adopting Hay principles: Greatly improved health; freedom from colds and catarrh; indigestion pain eliminated; great relief from tiredness and chronic sleeplessness; constipation a thing of the past; arthritic pain vanished or lessened greatly; relief from blinding headaches; disappearance of eczema and psoriasis; eradication of health-destroying allergies; effortless loss of excess weight; a clear complexion and shining head of hair. A number of people – including one 70-year-old lady – wrote to say that they were feeling well for the first time in their lives.

These letters provided convincing support for Dr Hay's argument that the *primary* cause of disease is not the outside germ, which always gets the blame, but the inside state of the body – the 'soil' – and that this is created mainly by wrong living habits and wrong eating habits.

It is of special interest, therefore, that in the middle of the nineteenth century, the famous French physiologist, Claude Bernard, argued similarly that health is best preserved by looking after *the terrain*, as he called it, and not by trying to eliminate disease-causing germs with the help of drugs. In a splendid article in *The Daily Telegraph* of 6 January 1993, the late Brian Inglis reminded us that Louis Pasteur (1822–95), the more famous French chemist and opponent of Bernard's theory, conceded on his death-bed that 'the germ is nothing . . . the terrain is everything.' Dr Hay could have no greater support for his argument than this.

The *Sunday Graphic* articles even brought Dr Hay post-haste to London from America. He contacted me immediately, asked me to dine with him, and expressed his approval of my articles. The upshot was that he asked me to write a book of menus and recipes for the British public. So I wrote *The Hay System Menu Book* (Harrap, 1937). Meanwhile, Dr Hay conducted a highly successful lecture tour throughout the UK. Before he returned to America he 'vetted' my book, gave it his blessing and wrote the foreword for it. He warned me that having written one book I would never be able to stop writing books! – and he made me his Public Relations Officer for Britain.

Dr Hay's prediction came true; I soon found myself writing a succession of books. *The Hay System Menu Book* was followed five years later by *Feeding the Family in Wartime*, written as part of my war work, with royalties donated to the Merchant Navy. Two years later (1944) Faber & Faber published *Your Daily Bread*, which started thousands of women everywhere successfully making their own 'no-kneading' whole-wheat bread. It also helped to inspire several noble Lords, including Hankey, Teviot and Sempill, to debate in 'the other place' the important issue of white versus wholewheat bread. I was present, by invitation of these same noble Lords, at several *very* lively debates!

During one debate (to which, on that occasion, I was listening from the 'Peeresses' Box'), I had a very amusing experience. One of the anti-wholewheat bread peers was claiming that wholewheat bread did not 'keep' at all well. This prompted the Lady on my left to lean towards me and whisper in my ear: 'What nonsense! My home-baked wholewheat bread keeps beautifully for eight or nine days!'. I whispered back, 'How do you make it?' The reply astonished me, 'I make it the Doris Grant way,' whereupon I confessed, 'I am Doris Grant – may I know to whom I have the pleasure of speaking?' She then told me (still in whispers) that she was Lady Hankey. It was Lord Hankey who, that day, had inaugurated the debate.

Sadly, I missed a subsequent debate on bread when, as members of his family delight to relate, Lord Hankey waved a Grant Loaf at the noble peers! *Your Daily Bread*, according to Hatchards bookshop in Piccadilly, became a steady seller for many years thereafter.

Ten years later, in 1954, I wrote *Dear Housewives*, about the dangers to health of devitalized, adulterated foodstuffs, and how to guard against them. Presentation copies of this book were sent to hundreds of schools and many universities throughout Britain, in the hope that it would prove a help and a guide to those responsible for the feeding of the young people in their care. This gift was made possible by the generosity of parents who were deeply concerned about the nutrition of their children at school and college, and by the offer of the author to forego royalties. The presentation copies were accompanied by an explanatory letter strongly recommending *Dear Housewives* and signed by (Lords) Douglas of Barloch, Hanky, Sempill, Teviot and Sir Robert McCarrison.*

Four years later, in 1958, I wrote *Housewives Beware*. I designed the dust jacket for this book, and the decorations throughout, as I also did for my three previous books. Then followed *Your Bread and Your Life*, a revised edition of *Your Daily Bread*, and *Your Daily Food: Recipe for Survival* in 1973, all published by Faber & Faber. An American edition of this latter book was published by Keats Publishing Inc. in 1974.

All my books up to this time contained, among other issues, Hay wisdom about food combining, and they brought a stream of letters containing remarkable accounts of benefits experienced. I did not write a book entirely devoted to food combining, however, until that published by Thorsons in 1984. Because of wartime and post-wartime food shortages and the wonder drug era, Dr Hay's message got somewhat lost. In any case, why bother to change your eating habits when there was 'a pill for every ill'? But from 1984 onwards *Food Combining for Health* proved dramatically that *'there is nothing so powerful as an idea whose time has come'*.

In 10 years, five editions of the book achieved a phenomenal 80 reprints, with sales of over half a million copies, and over 150 inclusions (to date) in *The Sunday Times* bestsellers lists. It has been translated

---

* School meals are still so unhealthy that in 1992 the Caroline Walker Trust, in association with the School Meals Campaign, published *National Guidelines for School Meals*, an expert report designed to encourage delicious and healthy meals in schools.

into seven foreign languages: Portuguese, Spanish, Greek, Hebrew, Serbo-Croat, Dutch and Finnish (and an eighth translation, for Korea, is now in the offing). It had become an international bestseller.

It all started in 1978, when I wrote a three-part article for *Healthy Living* magazine entitled 'Don't Mix Foods that Fight'. It was the tremendous response to this article that prompted the writing of *Food Combining for Health*, with Jean Joice as co-author. The title of the article was my own original slogan, and it became a very popular description of food combining in reviews and in a number of books on allied subjects. It was used by Thorsons, too, as a subtitle on one edition of our book. It also became the slogan for the Hay System Buffet which the Cumberland Hotel in London opened in their newly designed coffee shop. This buffet ran for several years, and was inspired by the publication of *Food Combining for Health*.

When Jean Joice and I wrote this book, we thought we knew all the remarkable things the Hay way of eating could do, but when the grateful letters began arriving thick and fast, we found we did not know the half of them! Readers wrote to say that the book had transformed their lives, quite often dramatically, and in some cases, it seems, they were convinced it had even rescued them from an early death.

Jean and I stress, however, as did Dr Hay himself, that it is not the Hay way of eating which achieves such miracles of healing – and of effortless slimming. Food combining merely boosts the body's own incredible but all-too-often-forgotten healing powers, *and allows the body to heal itself*.

Did my husband adopt the Hay System when I did?

No, and intentionally, he did not receive any urgings from me. He found no compelling reason to do so, and this is an indispensable ingredient for its successful adoption and enjoyment.

Fortunately, he loved all fruits and vegetables, especially our homegrown (organic) produce, and so his diet, although not completely 'Hay', was a very healthy one. Until he retired, his home-prepared meals helped considerably to counteract years of the usual, inevitably 'mixed-up' business lunches. When *Food Combining for Health* became a runaway bestseller, he gradually took on board, not all, but most of the Hay rules.

He is now 93 and looks younger than many men in their 70s. Shortly after his 92nd birthday, at his yearly medical examination for his car insurance policy, the doctor exclaimed: 'I can't find anything wrong with you – you are good for another 10 years!'

Incidentally, for many years my husband has been the sole baker in my house of 'the Grant loaf' – so called by friends and readers. He has adapted it to create his own version, known as 'the Gordon Grant loaf' – and excellent bread it is!

Finally, to conclude 'my own experience', I would like, briefly, to describe some of the leisure pursuits which I took up with great success, thanks to the remarkable energy I enjoyed on my Hay lifestyle.

When I was 40, I started having cello lessons. I found playing a cello utterly absorbing, and worked at it so enthusiastically that I was able to take the Grade V Associated Board of Music examination after only two years of lessons, gaining 'Distinction plus'. After six years at Watford School of Music, I won first prize for 'Senior Cello Playing'.

Some years later I became my husband's one and only crew on his 40-ft. motor-yacht; took navigation lessons, and did my share of 'setting a course' when cruising in the Channel Islands, up the Seine to Paris, or along the French coast from Cherbourg to St Malo. I was able, when cruising, to indulge my love of outdoor sketching.

I did a lot of pioneering work: crusading for the removal of the infamous 'agene' (a flour improver which caused health problems in humans and fits in dogs until eventually banned) from the nation's bread; and talking to Townswomen's Guilds, Church Guilds and Women's Institutes up and down the country, introducing them to the benefits of a wholefood larder, and especially to 100% whole-wheat, home-baked, 'no-kneading' bread. I also gave demonstrations on flower arranging – a very fascinating hobby.

My chief hobby, however, was designing and making costume jewellery. I had the honour of making many pieces for Norman Hartnell, the Queen's dress-maker, when he opened a boutique in his Bruton Street salon – and I had the great amusement of seeing his mannequins walking up and down at dress shows, wearing my brooch and earring sets!

Dr Hay wrote: 'When in splendid health every breath we draw is filled with inspiration, everything we do is full of interest, there are so many things to do, so much to accomplish . . . .' I am still proving, at 90, how true were his words.

Food Combining – It Works

When meditating over a disease I never think
of finding a remedy, but instead a means of
prevention.

(Louis Pasteur, 1884)

The success of food combining lies in the fact that it
is not a diet per se, but a most enjoyable and health-
giving lifestyle, based on the guiding principles
(known as the Hay System) that Dr William Howard
Hay (1866–1940), an American physician, began
teaching at the beginning of this century.

Briefly, the theory of the System is that protein
foods – meat, fish, poultry, cheese, etc. – and acid
fruits should not be eaten at the same meal with
starches – bread, potatoes, cereals, etc., and sugary
foods. This is Dr Hay's *Rule Number One*. His *Rule
Number Two* is that vegetables, salads and fruits should
form the major part of the diet. *Rule Number Three* is
that proteins and starches should be eaten in moderation. *Rule Number Four* is that only wholegrain and
unprocessed starches should be used, and all refined,
processed foods should be taboo – in particular, white

flour and sugar and all foods made with them; and all highly processed fats such as margarine and low fat spreads.

These are Dr Hay's main rules. A fifth one stipulates that an interval of at least four to five hours should elapse between meals of different character. Once learned, however, following these rules becomes surprisingly simple, almost second nature.

Without question they work – witness the extensive anecdotal evidence in Chapter 3. Many experts now agree that these rules '*seem* to work', but are unable to explain why or how. As a mere laywoman, I have dared to put forward what I feel to be a logical explanation later in this chapter.

Without question, also, is the tremendous popularity of this way of eating – a fact borne out by the sheer number of books on the subject which have been published worldwide during the past few years. But a number of these books contain departures from Dr Hay's principles which some would-be followers find confusing; they are somewhat stricter, particularly in the use of fruit. It should be emphasized, therefore, that *Food Combining for Health* is the original Hay guide.

Since the publication of *Food Combining for Health*, which fully explains the Hay system and how to put it into practice, there has been a constant stream of grateful letters from readers who have successfully overcome, or found relief from, many widely differing complaints – such as urticaria, migraine, duodenal ulcers, hay fever, asthma, allergies, overweight, the common cold, and many chronic conditions which appear to defeat the most complex medical theories and treatments.

There have been very few letters from people who did not benefit from the Hay System, and these cases, when examined, were mainly through not following the rules properly, or to too frequent but understandable 'cheating'.

Sceptics ask: 'How on earth can any diet, however good, cure so many different diseases?' The answer is simple. Food combining does not cure any disease – it merely allows the body to heal itself. As one reader wrote: 'I can see why many people cannot believe in food combining; it is so simple and effective, and quick, that the results sound too marvellous to be true!'

Nevertheless, an encouraging number of general practitioners do believe in it, are following it themselves and prescribing it for many patients – quite often with dramatic results. Many medical scientists and orthodox nutritionists still dismiss the cardinal rule – the starch/protein concept – as 'a load of rubbish'. But if the Hay system seems to work, that is all that matters. Case histories – many clinically confirmed by doctors and/or surgeons – are too numerous and too constant to be by chance, spontaneous regression, better food, or 'purely psychological'.

In his book, *A Doctor in the Wilderness*, Dr Walter Yellowlees, former president of the McCarrison Society, writes: 'In spite of dazzling advances in our understanding of physiology, there remain vast areas of our ignorance; this is true of the digestive processes and the cause or causes of food intolerance.'[1] Derek Bryce-Smith, Professor of Organic Chemistry at Reading University, and the brilliant campaigner for lead-free petrol and a lead-free environment, similarly admits: 'Once food enters the mouth a highly complicated process takes place. It is so very complicated that, even now, we are still learning what exactly happens.'[2]

How sad, therefore, that professional conservatism and scepticism have stifled any scientific curiosity as to WHY food combining seems to work so very successfully. This is, without doubt, preventing the relief of much suffering. As Derek Bryce-Smith bluntly points out: 'Professional conservatism is now proving a major obstacle to progress, thereby causing many patients to suffer unnecessarily as sacrifices to the altar of orthodoxy.'[2]

The Alkaline Medium

Hundreds of readers' letters received during the past 50 years of my writing life strongly suggest that food combining principles work and appear to relieve much unnecessary suffering. But medical sceptics find that the starch/protein concept is unacceptable, and argue that the alkaline medium, which Dr Hay stipulated is necessary for the preliminary digestion of starches, is impossible, as the stomach is always acid. Medical textbooks, however, teach that acidity rises as food is eaten. Moreover, McDowall's textbook on physiology states that *acidity rises higher when meat is eaten than when food consumed is bread.*[3]

The explanation could well be, therefore, that when meat and bread are eaten together, the extra acidity which accompanies the digestion of meat is sufficient

to neutralize the alkaline saliva which always impreg-
nates chewed food but which, according to Dr Hay,
is necessary *for the first 30 to 40 minutes* to prepare
the starches for subsequent digestion in the small
intestine.

In 1936, the work of three Philadelphia investigators provided near-indisputable confirmation of
the Hay System concept. In *Man Alive You're Half
Dead!*[4] Dr Daniel Munroe gives an account of a study
on five subjects by these investigators showing the
degree of acidity in the stomach after protein meals,
after starch meals, and after meals consisting of starch
and protein together. Their study revealed that 1½
hours after these meals were eaten, it was clear that in
the latter 'mixed' meal the proteins were being
digested under difficulties as the acidity present
was far lower than that shown as required by the
all-protein meal, and had been cut to one-third by
the presence of the starches and their accompanying
alkalies.

This investigation clearly showed that when the
concentrated starches and concentrated proteins are
mixed at one meal, there is too much acidity to permit
the continued reduction of the starch, and not enough
acid to cope sufficiently with the protein. The serious
implications of imperfectly digested proteins are
discussed later in this book.

The rightness of Dr Hay's concept was confirmed
at the beginning of the century by the work of the
famous Russian physiologist, Ivan Pavlov.[5] From his
celebrated observations on dogs, Pavlov deduced that
minced beef fed to a dog is digested in about four
hours, starch by itself is passed through a dog's

stomach in much less time, white bread more slowly than brown. But when meat was mixed with starch there was invariably delay – a protracted delay. Instead of about 4 hours for meat alone, this mixture took 8 hours or more to leave the stomach. In humans, delay in one section of the line tends towards delay all along the lines; this spells constipation. In a paper entitled 'Amylaceous Dyspepsia' in *The Liverpool Medico-Chirurgical Journal* (1931), Dr Lionel Picton (of Cheshire Testament fame), confirmed that meals of mixed character, such as meat and bread, favour constipation, whereas meat and salad at one meal and starch, such as bread and butter, at a separate meal, have no such effect. Dr Picton's paper (on starch-related indigestion) provided yet more support for the starch/protein concept – as did the case histories of his patients.

It is of special significance, in view of Pavlov's observations on dogs, that Jean Joice and I receive frequent reports from food combining followers who are feeding their dogs biscuits at one meal and meat at a separate meal – with excellent results. One amusing report concerned a doctor who possessed an obvious flare for scientific investigation. He decided to 'try it on the dog'. His retriever suffered from distressing diarrhoeas and had a most unsocial habit of letting off foul stinks in the living room. The experiment was a success. In no time the diarrhoeas improved greatly and the stinks abated. Other reports received concerned dogs recovering from arthritis – one dog even losing his arthritic limp and recovering his enthusiasm for 'walkies'.

It is not surprising, therefore, that there have been

many letters from arthritic sufferers. Mixed meals
appear to be among the chief contributors to certain
forms of arthritis and allied conditions. This can be
partly explained by the evidence that when starches
and sugars are eaten with meat and other proteins at
the same meal, the former decompose and create acids
which can then induce a form of acid intoxication. The
chief acid so produced is that known as oxalic acid.[6]

It is an interesting fact that dogs developed marked
oxalic poisoning when fed meat and sugar at the same
meal – despite both meat and sugar being free from
oxalic acid. In *Natural Health, Sugar and the Criminal
Mind*, J. I. Rodale points out: 'This oxalic acid when it
reaches the blood converts soluble lime salts into an
insoluble oxalate of lime, and this induces the condition of the system known as decalcification, or lime
starvation.'[6] This condition is conducive to various
types of rheumatism, and contributes to osteoporosis.
Properly combined meals, on the other hand, which
avoid mixtures of starch and sugar with meat and other
proteins, not only prevent the production of oxalic acid
but liberate the calcium (lime) in the diet for the vital
work of building strong bones and teeth, giving tone to
the muscles and stability to the nerves.

Incompletely Digested Proteins

Properly combined meals also prevent the formation of
incompletely digested proteins. This is important, as
these split up into intermediate or large protein molecules that are toxic. Some of these toxic proteins are
known to cause immune reactions and be responsible

for many common allergies such as hay fever, asthma, eczema, urticaria and migraine.[4]

In view of Dr Hay's warnings of harm from *incompletely digested proteins*, the research findings of Dr Nadya Coates, scientist and cancer specialist, are of special interest. She found that permeability of the gut caused by fungal candida enables *inadequately digested particles of food* to be transplanted into the bloodstream, and 'is one of the major contributing factors in the undermining of the body's defence system – an undermining which if not arrested could ultimately result in serious disease.'[7]

In a letter to *The Lancet*, 27 March 1976, Dr W. A. Hemmings drew attention to the possible role in human disease of incompletely digested proteins. He wrote: 'It has been known since the first decade of this century that small quantities of dietary protein are absorbed from the gut in sufficient amounts to give rise to immune reaction. However, we have shown that much larger quantities of dietary protein are absorbed into the circulation after only *partial cleavage* [added emphasis] of the molecules.' He questioned the toxicological significance of these incompletely broken down proteins as well as their 'logical role in human disease'.*

---

* According to a press report in February 1995, researchers at the Bristol Royal Infirmary have found (in the largest study of its kind) higher-than-normal levels of dietary protein in the blood of osteoarthritis patients. Their findings, which are to be published in British and American medical journals, appear to provide strong confirmation of Dr Hemmings' fears regarding the possible role in human disease of incompletely digested proteins which have been absorbed into the bloodstream. Their findings, moreover, also appear to provide excellent vindication of Dr Hay's starch/protein rule which *prevents* the formation of these harmful proteins.

The importance of Dr Hay's starch/protein rule, especially where allergies are concerned, lies in the fact that it prevents the formation of incompletely digested proteins, which are thought to encourage the growth of germs or 'moulds' or viruses. Imperfectly synthesized protein – which can arise from unnaturally speeding up the growth of factory-farmed animals for earlier marketing – is also thought to encourage the growth of germs or viruses. This is a serious aspect of factory-farming that has been lamentably overlooked by the health ministries, but it could well shed light on the serious epidemics of diseases to which factory-farmed animals and birds are now susceptible.

That these facts have been overlooked by the medical and agricultural scientists is most likely because of the still prevailing but now outmoded 'germ theory' of disease.[8] This postulates that the germ or virus is the *primary* cause of disease and always as *an exogenous factor* (arising from without). Medical scientists, however, are now discovering that the germ or virus can be *an endogenous factor* (arising from within) and, moreover, that disease can in fact develop *from viruses or bacteria carried, usually harmlessly, by the host.*[9]

Dr Luria, a virologist of international reputation writes: 'A new view of the nature of viruses is emerging. They used to be thought of solely as foreign intruders – strangers to the cells they invade or parasitize. But recent findings, including the discovery of a host-induced modification of viruses, emphasize more and more the similarity of viruses to hereditary units such as genes. Indeed, some viruses are being considered as bits of heredity in search of a chromosome.'[10]

In 1942, in a letter to *The Times*, another view of the nature of viruses was suggested by J.E.R. MacDonagh, Hunterian Professor of The Royal College of Surgeons in London – that viruses should not be regarded as a cause of infectious illness but as its consequence – the consequence of a breakdown in the body's defence mechanisms.

A distinguished French scientist, Professor André Voisin, discussed yet another concept of the virus in his book *Soil, Grass and Cancer*.[11] He pointed out that under certain conditions the nucleo-protein of the cell can be transformed to the virus molecule, and quotes supporting research by a Japanese scientist, Yamafugi, and his colleagues.[12] This research has shown how a disturbance of the metabolism can cause this transformation.

Nutrition, therefore, could possibly be the whole crux of the matter.

Whether defective proteins or defective 'rogue' genes will cause harm, or not, may depend on the state of the body soil – *the terrain*. In other words, this will depend on faulty or good nutrition. It is comforting to know that a genetic predisposition to disease – to cancer for instance – does not mean that it is inevitable. In the Winter 1933 *Newsletter* of the World Cancer Research Fund, the Editor writes: 'It is not necessarily our genes that give us cancer but the behaviour of those genes in our bodies, and outside factors like the food we eat can play a very large role in regulating how genes can act.'

In the early years of this century, Sir Albert Howard, distinguished agricultural scientist and pioneer of organic farming and gardening, tumbled to the connection between improperly synthesized or digested proteins and virus disease during his work at the Research Institute at Pusa in Bengal. He wrote: 'Foot-and-mouth disease is considered to be a virus disease. It could be more correctly described as *a simple consequence of malnutrition* [added emphasis], due to the fact that the proteins have not been properly synthesized, or to some obvious error of management.'[13] During his work in Pusa, he several times observed with keen interest his healthy, well-fed and 'innoculation-free' oxen rubbing noses over a low hedge with foot-and-mouth infected cases. *Nothing happened.* His animals failed to react to the disease.

Had Howard's observations received the attention they merited, 'much of the confusion over disease correctly or incorrectly ascribed to viruses ... might have been dispelled.' So concluded Dr Morton Biskind, noted American virologist.[14]

There is now deep concern among farmers and the public – especially among those buying, or not buying, meat for their families – about the increasing prevalence in cattle of BSE ('mad cow disease'). According to a report in *The Mail on Sunday* in September 1994, there may well be a connection between 'mad cow disease' and *improperly synthesized proteins.* In reply to a question 'What is BSE?', Keith Meldrum, Chief Veterinary Officer for the Agriculture Ministry, replied that no one really knows the exact nature of BSE. He did, however, stress the fact that the infectious agents were not bacteria or viruses: 'It's believed,' he replied, 'to be spread by a "deformed" protein called a prion. Prions, new to science, reproduce by tipping normal proteins in the host animal into the shape which can cause disease. Unlike other forms of life, they do not contain DNA. Prions are responsible for all the transmissible spongiform encephalopathies. These include BSE, CJD in humans and scrapie in sheep.'

The question therefore arises: if a deformed protein (a 'prion') is the same as, or similar to, an incompletely digested or synthesized protein, then the incorporation until recently of animal proteins in the feeding stuffs of cattle and poultry may have been a major cause of BSE and salmonella. Cattle and poultry are *herbivores*, and as such are not constitutionally capable of properly digesting *animal proteins*.

BSE in cattle, and salmonella in poultry, might therefore both be explained by Sir Albert Howard's conclusion regarding foot-and-mouth disease – '*A simple consequence of malnutrition.*' If so, Dr Hay was many years ahead of his time when he warned of the possible serious effects of incompletely digested proteins ('prions'?) on humans.

These facts shed entirely new light on the importance and validity of Dr Hay's starch/protein concept – his *rule number one* – which helps to ensure properly digested proteins. Moreover, they clearly demolish the widely-held belief that the tendency to develop this or that disease is because of the genes inherited from our parents, hence nothing helpful can be done about it. Dr Hay was convinced that heredity is not to blame, and 'that on our parents we may blame only our predisposition to disease of this or that organ, the actual disease being always a thing of our own creation.'

As recently as the 1960s and 1970s, doctors, too,

believed that our medical destiny was based on heredity and that nothing much could be done about it. Moreover, they derided nutrition as a therapy and regarded any physician who prescribed vitamins and good nutrition as a 'quack'. In fact, in medical schools after World War II, the advocacy of health-giving food was seen to be the raving of cranks.[1]

Now, however, in the 1980s and early 1990s, there has been much evidence of a change in medical thinking; many medical authorities are now urging a switch in emphasis from 'curative' medicine to 'preventative' medicine, giving priority to nutrition. This is clearly evident in publications such as the World Health Organisation's latest report, *Diet, Nutrition and the Prevention of Chronic Diseases*. In this report, WHO strongly supports the view: 'That a number of chronic diseases can be prevented to a substantial extent by lifestyle changes, among which diet plays a crucial role.'[15]

It is highly significant in this respect, according to an article in *The Sunday Times* of 21 January 1993, that in January of that year doctors began a £9m Europe-wide investigation of links between diet and cancer.

The Importance of the Chemical Balance

In the correct chemical balance of the 'bodysoil' – *the terrain* – lies the secret of optimum health. In order to attain this, Dr Hay recommended that the major part of the diet should consist of fresh vegetables, salads and fruits – his *rule number two*. These foods are of vital importance, being classed as alkaline-forming:

when metabolized they leave behind what Dr Hay termed an 'alkaline ash' – a meaningless term for orthodox scientists and nutritionists. But Dr Hay regarded this alkaline ash as the vital part of the food, and claimed that textbooks on nutrition paid no attention to its high significance as a possible essential for the maintenance of the correct chemical balance. This, in a healthy body, should be approximately four parts alkaline to one part acid. When the body approaches this ideal the immune system becomes more efficient, as evidenced by the freedom from infections and astonishing freedom from colds which well-established Hay followers invariably experience.

The effects of Dr Hay's 'alkaline ash' could possibly be similar to those of today's much publicized antioxidants, protecting and boosting the immune system in particular. An efficient immune system is more than ever important in this present age. Chronic diseases have increased in the last two decades, and an increasingly polluted environment is putting an added burden on our greatly overworked immune systems. (How unforgivably irresponsible, therefore, that our health departments are still promoting the addition of a potent pollutant – fluoride – to our already polluted drinking water and one, moreover, that may well depress the immune system, according to the research of Dr Sheila Gibson.[16]

Dr Hay's claim that the secret of health lies in the chemical balance of the body was made as long ago as the 1930s, but it was derided by the doctors of his day. Now, over 60 years later, a number of scientists are proving him right – so very right.

According to recent research, eating a high

proportion of alkaline-forming foods (vegetables, salads, fruits) is highly beneficial to both physical and mental health (*rule number two*). It lessens the incidence of some types of arthritis, encourages youthful vitality, and discourages aggressive behaviour. The well-known American criminologist, Alexander Schauss,found the alkaline-acid balance of the diet a vital factorwhen working with delinquents and criminals.[17] Psychologist Stanley Shachter, Department of Psychology, Columbia University, New York, found that people smoked less when their alkaline-acid balance is good.[18] What a pity this is not known by smokers who genuinely want to give up smoking!

And, psychologist and nutritionist Patrick Holford, Director of the Institute of Optimum Nutrition, revealed that unexplained aches and pains, strange cravings and moods, can result from a deficiency of alkaline-producing foods in the diet.[19]

On the other hand, according to author Celia Wright, a high proportion of these foods in the diet produces a tremendous sense of well-being, as well as calmness, emotional stability, strength without aggression, and a feeling of constant optimism.[20]

Rules number three and four of the Hay System are also of great importance. They, too, help to boost the immune system: By reducing the intake of acid-forming proteins and starches (*rule number three*), and by cutting out refined processed foods, especially white flour and sugar, and using 'whole' foods instead (*rule number four*).

The Hay System, apart from the starch/protein rule is, therefore, virtually the same wholefood diet promoted some twelve years ago by the Royal College of Physicians, and some eight years ago by the World Health Organisation's report: *Diet, Nutrition and the Prevention of Chronic Diseases.*[15]

The countless tributes from Hay System followers strongly suggest not only that food combining works successfully, but *in a way which no other diet can do*.

3

Success

> The proof of the pudding is in the eating thereof.

Dr Hay wrote: 'It has been a marvellous intelligence that has created so perfect a machine as man, and no matter what name we call this intelligence, its supreme wisdom enlists our awe.'

During the 10 years since the publication of *Food Combining for Health* its authors have received countless letters from Hay System followers and have been privileged to witness, through these letters, remarkable healings brought about by this 'supreme wisdom' when operating with a properly combined diet.

How sad, therefore, that there are millions of people whose chronic diseases are not being healed or prevented by conventional medicine. As Dr Chris Thompson and Dr Dennis MacEoin state in *The Health Crisis* (The Natural Medicines Society): 'Regrettably, conventional medicine is only belatedly moving towards causative principles, but even in this area there is a serious reluctance to recognize the crucial role of diet.'

Dr Hay regarded every illness, acute or chronic, as 'merely the effort of the body to clean house and right its internal discord'. Correctly combining the food we eat, is by far the simplest, cheapest, and most successful way of righting this discord. Celia Wright firmly agrees. In *The Wright Diet* she states: '. . . sorting out your food combinations can be the blessing you've been waiting for. I've known people for whom this method was the only one, from everything that nutritional healing has to offer, that worked for them.'

The remarkable case histories and extracts from readers' letters included in this chapter bear witness to this. They are all genuine and have been received by me over the years. I decided not to include people's names in order to preserve confidentiality.

Some years ago, as part of a promotional scheme, my publishers decided to use some of these extracts as testimonials. After choosing them from a broad selection, the extracts were enlarged, arranged on a display board and reproduced for representatives to place in bookshops and health stores. The reps were impressed – but one, with uncharacteristic scepticism, thought they were too good to be true, and was convinced that the extracts were made up. They were not, of course, but this story serves to show how almost unbelievable can seem the benefits that may result from following the Hay System.

Enjoyment in Eating

This system, however, is not only highly beneficial, it is also a very enjoyable way of eating for health, as the following excerpts reveal. Moreover, it does not preclude gourmet cooking.

'We have almost completed a week on the Hay System, and have found it wonderful in every way. I am really enjoying preparing and eating the meals. Not one grumble from Edwin yet! And the bonus for me is the termination of indigestion; it really does work, not mixing foods that fight.'

'I'm still on the Hay diet, after three years! I can't imagine that I will ever want to eat any other way now. I have no arthritis twinges, which is wonderful, and I have plenty of energy, which amazes me as teaching at the moment is very demanding.'

'I do thank you for your invaluable work that has kept my family well and happy, and all those recipes that make cooking an interesting adventure and not to have to ask "*What on earth can I cook today?*" '

'It is just a year since I became a devotee of food combining, and it continues to be a source of inspiration in my life. Contemporaries some-times tell me that they lose interest in cooking, living alone. This does not happen to me and *I enjoy all that I eat* and can say the challenge has added interest to my life where there was dire need.'

'My pleasure in food has increased as pain and discomfort has ceased.

'My husband, too, enjoys the many and various raw salads with which we invariably begin each meal when at home. They are a continuing joy, and we would never want to return to our old modus vivendi.'

'Like many people with good intentions, I had been mostly eating the correct items, but not in the right sequence or combinations. After the first day, my mental clarity increased. After the second day, my stomach became much flatter and more comfortable. I had lost the urge to drink instant coffee, and was feeling much younger (i.e. 45 feeling more like 25). Some minor stiffness in my hips and lower back has left me. *All these benefits, and still eating sumptuous meals!* I will certainly promote it to friends as well as giving it its due place in my thesis write up.' (The thesis was for a degree at the Department of Geography and Environmental Studies, University of Tasmania.)

'I had roast chicken with roasted root vegetables, boiled peas with a little soured cream dressing – tangerines to start with and orange sections with

cream to finish . . . I sat down to a meal – tho' I
say it to myself – fit for a king!'

The Speed with which Benefits
Become Apparent

Would-be food combiners frequently ask 'how long
will it take to experience results?' This can depend on
how chronic are the symptoms, but many new arrivals
on the Hay scene have been astonished at the remarkable speed with which their symptoms were banished
or ameliorated.

'Thank you for your wonderful food combining
book which my homoeopath referred me to for
help with arthritis. I stopped limping *within a
week* and the stabbing pain which made me
scream stopped within two.'

'For the past three months I have been following
the advice in *Food Combining for Health*, and was
delighted when I lost my life-long acid stomach
after the first meal. Constipation and arthritic
pains are also under control.'

'After the first week, severe indigestion had
almost completely gone, and now, 17 weeks later,
a factor I have almost forgotten about.'

'For years I have been plagued with an allergy and
slight asthma. The allergy resembled urticaria,
only worse. I was covered from head to toe with

giant hives, swelling of eyelids, lips and throat. I resembled "a boxer after a fight", only I had no bruises. I have tried doctors, drugs, dermatologists, homoeopathy, acupuncture and herbalism in that order with no lasting effect.

'Two weeks before Christmas a friend asked me to read your book and see what I thought of it. I had nothing to lose at this stage. I was beginning to despair. I recently had a urine test which showed a very high ratio of acid. On reading the part in your book referring to acid convinced me at least to try the diet.

'*I really couldn't believe it but within four days the rash had gone.* It was wonderful to be able to eat foods that for years had been denied me. Christmas was also wonderful. The pudding and turkey stuffing (both compatible recipes) were delicious and I did not feel in any way deprived. I could even have a "drink".'

'I am happy to tell you that I am among the many who feel your book has changed their lives. The greatest surprise has been how quickly the beneficial effects of the diet have become apparent – less than two months in my case.'

'I lost two pounds in weight in one week without even trying or being hungry.'

'As you no doubt have heard many times, I felt very much better after only two weeks.'

'Now, since I've had two days of compatible eating my guts do not blow up to the same extent.'

'I have been on the Hay System for the past three weeks and I have slept soundly every night *for the first time in nearly 20 years.*'

'After a week on the Hay System, I was able to walk without a wheelchair.'

'I had 36 hours of withdrawal symptoms for some strange reason – nausea, headaches and general feeling of unwellness. On *the afternoon of the second day* I started to feel better, and from then on felt terrific.'

(Withdrawal symptoms on starting food combining are experienced by some people. These symptoms can be caused by a release of toxins from the body, such as are experienced sometimes at the beginning of a fruit fast, or giving up an addiction such as chocolate or alcohol.)

Indigestion, Ulcers and Constipation

A very large number of letters received have been from victims of chronic indigestion. In many cases relief has been virtually instant and quite dramatic.

It is of special interest to food combiners that Dr Kenneth Vickery, distinguished lifetime crusader for healthy food and Vice-President of The Royal Institute of Public Health, wrote of constipation: 'In contrast to the inoffensive stools of wildlife subsisting on natural food, the malodorous stools of man are indicative of a sophisticated, unhealthy diet – typically excess sugar in the presence of protein.' – an unhealthy mixture avoided by Dr Hay's starch/protein rule.

'I started using the Hay System two months ago having had a digestive problem for the last 10 years since having a hysterectomy. I have become very anaemic (blood count four) and it took me a long time to regain my strength. I have had an increasing problem digesting starch but never knew what I was doing wrong . . . . I was very depressed and unable to cope. When I bought your book I was overjoyed, at last I understood the problem, and I set to with great excitement. *The results were miraculous.* The pains which had been increasing in number in my hands and finger joints went, and a wonderful feeling of calm settled over me. I felt able to cope, happy and more energetic . . . .'

'I recently saw a young man who was crippled with stomach pain and heart burn. He was taking all sorts of digestive cures from his doctor, and becoming very restricted in what he could eat. In a couple of weeks of the Hay System he was back to normal, working with a very stressful job, and eating every type of food as long as it was in the right order. He phones me regularly to thank me for the system.'

'Recently met a retired naval chap – invalided out of the navy because of digestive upsets – miraculous recovery after reading *Food Combining* . . . .'

'For the past year I have been following Dr Hay's system, using *Food Combining for Health* as my basis. I have been amazed to experience pain-free digestion and elimination *for the first time in my life*, despite the fact that I have studied nutrition for many years and have applied these studies to my diet.'

'I am writing to thank you very much for writing your great book, *Food Combining for Health* and thereby helping to introduce this great, cheap and effective health system to thousands of people like me.

'I was on the verge of being killed by constipation from which I had been suffering for the past 21 years. It miraculously went away on the third day of my fruit fasting, even before I had begun the Hay System proper.

'I have introduced more than 50 people who

are now practising faithfuls. I couldn't wait for them to ask about it and I thought no one should be denied a knowledge of it just on account of prejudice. In some cases, however, especially with orthodox doctors, I met bias and resistance in acceptance of the almost unbelievable powers of this system. But all resistance usually melted after I reluctantly lent your book to them. The idea is now spreading like bush fire as those introduced introduce others. And, in addition, there is also the fact that people have been disillusioned with orthodox Western medicine and are looking for any alternative that works.

'I am a journalist with a background in science. I wonder whether the only help I can render to this great system is just by popularizing your book. I wish I could do more but I don't know how.'

'I have a copy of your book *Food Combining for Health* and have been following the diet for about 10 months.

'I have been very pleased with the results. The benefits being freedom from constipation, coughs, colds and sore throats. I have suffered from constant sore throats all my life and haven't had a single one since beginning the diet. . .

'It has long puzzled me why people who keep themselves fit and eat "healthy food" still get colds and flu. My own experience with the Hay diet in keeping me free from those illnesses for nearly a year now has shown me that it doesn't matter how much exercise you do or how much "health food" you eat, if you don't combine foods properly you are wasting your time. I wish I had found your book a long time ago when my children were small – how much healthier we all would have been.'

A doctor writes:

'I am having great success with patients for whom I have prescribed compatible eating. One patient had been plagued with indigestion for over 20 years. In less than a week she was completely free of pain. Another patient had been badly constipated for many years. When she turned up at a recent surgery complaining that she was still constipated despite the whole-food diet with extra bran on which she had been living for the past four years, I advised her to try compatible eating with the help of *Food Combining for Health*. A week later she reported that her constipation had completely cleared.'

Weight Loss

Loss of excess weight – on average about 2 lb a week – is frequently reported as a totally unexpected and welcome bonus, achieved moreover while eating good amounts of food at each meal, even those foods usually regarded as fattening, such as potatoes, butter and cream.

According to many reports Jean and I have received from Hay System followers, merely avoiding mixtures of starch and protein and starch and acid fruits, is sufficient gradually to reduce excess weight *without even trying, without feeling hungry, without wearisome calorie counting, and without resorting to crash diets, appetite suppressants, or dangerous fat-reducing drugs.* Dr Hay warned that all fat-reducing drugs should be avoided as you would the plague; most of them have unpleasant, even dangerous, side-effects.

Obesity is a far more serious condition than most people realize; it is now closely linked with diabetes, cholesterol-rich gallstones and coronary artery disease. It is a matter of concern that nearly half the people in this country are overweight, and obesity in children is now reaching epidemic proportions.

When some slimming diets are discontinued, the excess weight rolls back again. Slimming the Hay way is not only effortless but the results are permanent.

'My husband has been wonderful – joining me in the early weeks, with the result that he has lost 21 lb., and I, too, am now 8 stone 5 lb. from 10 stone 6 lb. It was effortless.'

Peter Scudamore, eight times champion National Hunt jockey, had to battle all his working life to keep his weight down to 9 stone 12 lb. In a newspaper interview he reports:

'I was recommended the Hay diet when I visited a health farm. Before that I used to just skip meals and starve myself to keep the weight off, even though I knew how bad that is for your health. I feel so much better now I'm dieting properly, and I don't get nearly so tired. On a normal day I might have a melon for breakfast, a salad sandwich for lunch and some sort of protein and vegetables at night. It's such an easy programme to stick to. On Christmas Day, I had the same turkey and vegetables as my family, only I didn't have any starch or potatoes.'

'I am feeling thrilled with myself because I read your book *Food Combining for Health*, and three months ago decided to try eating the right food combinations.

'Oh! What a wonderful treat, at last I have found the right foods that don't add weight but reduce it. The awful bulk fat I had put on over the years. Now friends comment on how well I look and are surprised to see how I have lost so much weight in such a short time. I have tried so many diets before, but *nothing has worked like this*. I can sit down, enjoy my meals and know that I am not going to put the size I was back again. My grateful thanks.'

'I have been eating by the Hay System for seven months now and do not intend to alter to my old ways. Taking the advice you gave me about not telling people about the diet I have been surprised by the number of people who have asked how I have lost so much weight. These include the local fishmonger, whose wife asked immediately for details of the book [*Food Combining for Health*] and intends to put her husband on the diet as soon as possible.

'Apart from the absence of my aches and pains I think the greatest boon for me is that I no longer suffer from almost constant hunger and could only keep going by having constant snacks.'

'Although not really overweight, it has been a joy to see the extra pounds disappear so quickly. Alas, not very long ago I was an emotional roller coaster, experiencing extreme highs and lows and was on the verge of asking for medical help. What a blessing I have found such a simple and natural cure for this problem. I'm now on a wonderfully 'even keel' and suddenly have more energy than I've had in years. Seem to have said goodbye to chronic insomnia as well. We have also become acutely aware of just how few people recognize the importance of what they eat and how many medical problems could be solved with a simple change in diet. We have changed our Great Dane's diet according to the Hay System and it seems to suit him very well – far better appetite and far less flatulence!'

'John is 50. A friend lent him your book *Food Combining for Health* ... he began following it and finds it quite remarkable. *He feels so well.* Initially he lost some weight but has now stabilized – and he thinks it is wonderful.'

Arthritis and Allied Conditions

There is a firm belief, both lay and medical, that no cure is available for arthritis, either osteo or rheumatoid, both of which can be completely disabling. It is the latter type which affects the younger person, but it is more often found in people between the ages of 30 to 35. The usual treatment is with analgesic painkillers and anti-inflammatory drugs which can ease symptoms, but which can also cause severe side-effects – as proved so tragically with the drug Opren, withdrawn from use over 13 years ago.

Although arthritis is the least amenable to treatment of all the chronic diseases, Dr Hay maintained that it responds to nutritional treatment as surely as do other degenerative diseases; that it can do so even if the pain seems to inhibit motion completely, provided, at the same time, that the joint can be moved passively to any degree. Tributes and case histories received from Hay devotees prove the truth of Dr Hay's words.

The following tribute appeared in *The Health Express* (Summer 1987). Donald Jennings, then 65, was a retired army driving instructor at Aldershot. His GP had diagnosed arthritis, and both his doctor and chiropractor had confirmed they couldn't help him very much:

'I now eat as much as I like and have still lost weight. I no longer count calories. Incredibly, in less than a month, I began to feel a definite improvement – I could sit without getting stiff, I could turn my head when reversing a car, I could sleep on my side at night and even my morning headaches of 10 years standing have gone.

'All this by a style of eating and no drugs at all. Another side-effect is that receding gums seem to have disappeared. Overall, it has been a magic cure for me – a way of eating that can virtually eliminate arthritis and associated headaches; cure sensitive teeth, lose *excess* fat and help skin conditions must be good. Worth a try I should say.'

'I have had slight attacks of arthritis since 1975. However, a recent attack starting around Christmas 1985 was more of an onslaught in its intensity. The pain, which was so excruciating that at times I was screaming, eventually attacked my whole body.

'It started with my feet and ankles, then legs and hips, hands, arms, spine and neck. I could not wear *any* of my own shoes or slippers, and eventually bought some slippers two or three sizes larger which I even wore when I went out! The swelling was incredible and my skin was taut and shiny.

'Treatment consisted of various painkillers and anti-inflammatory drugs. There were some days when I could not stand at all, and others when I walked, it felt like walking on RED HOT

GOLF BALLS. On top of this my circulation became very poor and several fingers and toes went "dead".

'By now I was wondering if I could ever walk again properly, let alone dance or drive an ordinary car. I was even considering a wheelchair and a walking frame. Then suddenly one day a great friend advised me to buy *Food Combining for Health*. I did, studied it carefully, started eating as advised, and within two or three days the pain and swelling started to subside. Within a month or so most of me was nearly back to normal. I was able to start driving again, which I love, and to dance again.

'To be out of that agony and to be mobile again and to have pain-free nights is something I shall be grateful for, for the rest of my life. I must add that the mental and emotional benefits from this new way of eating are quite extraordinary. I am able to think much more clearly and see problems through. Emotionally I am far steadier and calmer. Moreover, drinking alcohol seems to have lost its attraction. In fact I hardly ever seem to want to drink at all now, whereas I was quite fond of it before. I think this is *an extremely interesting and important 'side-effect' of eating this way.*'

'Within a week of starting Hay I was able to put a foot down without being startled into screaming by the pain. After the second week I wasn't even wincing, and I hung up my stick in the shed. After the third week I was walking normally. By the end of the summer I could run, jump, dance, turn cartwheels.'

'I have stuck rigidly to *Food Combining for Health* for the last three years and now, at 75, have acquired a bicycle, which is the joy of my life, especially riding by the sea in the early morning. Never have I felt so well.'

In a second letter this same correspondent writes:

'Considerable difficulties have arisen during the last year, to which, at long last, I believe I have said goodbye! However, I have not allowed anything to interfere with my food combining, and never shall, and my gratitude for the book will never lessen. *And* my cycling continues unabated!'

'A Poole woman with severe arthritis in her neck was put on to a neck brace by her doctor and told she would have to wear it for a very long time. Within two weeks of adopting compatible eating she was able to leave it off – except in bed at night. She is also feeling so much better in herself.'

'I must confess that I feel a great deal better. My arthritis, touch wood, has all but disappeared, and I have lost some of my surplus weight.'

'I bought *Food Combining for Health*, read it twice but did not practise its recommendations until two weeks later, when I developed crippling pains in my knees. After about 10 days on the food combining system the pain gradually alleviated. Now I've sent for the cookbook by Erwina Lidolt.'

'I was crippled with a form of ankylosing spondylitis (a type of arthritis) which attacked my feet and left knee. Not wishing to be beaten by the disease I started studying different diets and how their application can assist in recovery. A dear friend brought my attention to the Hay diet which I then followed as closely as I was able, and this, plus the care of a super doctor and enough strength of mind to refuse defeat, led to my eventual complete return to good health – and this after being told by my specialist that the arthritis might never leave me and I could end up unable to work or even walk properly again!'

'My brother in Morocco has just told me on the phone that people in Morocco who have arthritis are walking out of their wheelchairs!' [This is as a result of *Food Combining for Health*.]

'The joy when I woke up one morning and found I could actually move my thumb, and watch during the following week the awful swelling slowly die down and the pains dwindling. It was really a miracle.'

'After an accident dancing some years ago I developed arthritis of the spine and hip quite

badly, which gradually spread to other parts of
the body and I suffered for about eight years.
Finally I had a very bad attack and was unable to
walk, or even to turn over in bed. The doctor
prescribed very powerful painkillers and I
was eventually able to hobble around albeit still
in a lot of pain. It was at that point that I was
given a copy of *Food Combining for Health*, and
after following the Hay System for exactly one
month I found that all the pain had gone from
my spine, hip, shoulder, foot etc. . . . The book
has certainly been my saviour.'

'I am yet more proof that the Hay diet is
wondrous in its healing powers.

'I started the Hay diet in September last year.
At that time I had osteoarthritis in both hips, and
what was diagnosed as polyarthralgia – multiple
arthritic pain in every joint except my elbows,
inflamed wrists, knees and ankles – no power at
all in my wrists, and a left shoulder which was
completely locked. I was in constant pain day and
night, despite 150mg daily of Voltarol, shooting
pains in arms, hands and wrists. I never had a full
night's sleep – whenever I turned over the pain
woke me. I could only work in the mornings and
slept every afternoon for one-and-a-half to two
hours propped against the back of a couch. I
was totally exhausted by the pain, and unable to
do simple household chores or get into or out of
a bath.

'After a starch lunch and a protein dinner on
16 September 1994, I spent an evening with

hardly any pain. I slept all through that night. The next day I had a starch breakfast, an alkaline lunch and a protein dinner. I had much more energy all day and very little pain.

'Six weeks later I could reduce the dose of painkillers to one a day (which I still take). By 17 November 1994 I had lost half a stone in weight and noticed several other improvements: cellulite was vanishing, teeth were less sensitive, my ulcer was less sore and patches of eczema were clearing up.

'I visited a physiotherapist regularly to help my locked shoulder – she gave me exercises and acupuncture. I also attended the Homoeopathic Hospital out-patients department here in Glasgow and they prescribed for me. But still the Hay diet ruled whether or not I was in pain – if I strayed from it I suffered for it!

'Now in April 1995 I am still on the Hay diet, enjoying it enormously, and the pain is reduced almost to the level of discomfort. The E.S.R. rate of 57 has dropped to 25. I have *almost* full movement in my shoulder. My weight has dropped by more than a stone and stabilized. I still get tired, but I am working three full days a week and some extra hours, and I can contemplate once more some of the activities I used to enjoy like walking and bird-watching. I plan to start a t'ai chi exercise class in May to help build stamina.

'I still re-read *Food Combining for Health* and am constantly inspired by it. This is to say thank you. A year ago I thought I couldn't go on living. Now I feel I have a future.'

Jackie Le Tissier was only 22, full of the joys and challenges of life, when, over a period of months, she became progressively stricken with burning and crippling pains in her feet which, later, progressed to her left knee, along with swelling to such an extent that her feet almost doubled in size, making her look like Mickey Mouse from the knees down!:

'I have never experienced such physical distress before, and imagine my feeling of insult, on consulting a doctor, to be told to change my style of footwear! – knowing full well that the shoes I wore were in no way contributory to such acute discomfort.

'Needless to say the pain did not lessen. After several visits to another doctor I was eventually sent for blood tests. These indicated that I was suffering from an inflammatory condition. Anti-inflammatory medication was prescribed, which, although having an initial effect in reducing the pain, soon wore off, resulting in repeat prescriptions – but for stronger drugs.

'The intensity of the pain at this time was such that I admit to being reduced to tears on several occasions, and literally crawling upstairs on hands and knees, rather than having to suffer the agony of standing up.

'As the symptoms worsened so the drug doses changed and increased until I was referred to a specialist in an attempt to discover the nature of my affliction. It was then that the diagnosis of a form of ankylosing spondylitis – an arthritic condition – was made . . . . My relief at finally discovering what was wrong was soon dispelled, however, when prognosis was made. I was told that I might never be wholly well enough to maintain full-term employment, and might even end up in a wheelchair . . . .

'I had by now been forced to give up my job and return home to convalesce, making intermittent trips back to the specialist . . . . Drug treatment continued, but it was in 1984, following intense study of alternative "diets", and my determination to rid myself of medication, that a friend suggested I read her copy of the then recently published *Food Combining for Health*.

'Less than 12 months later I was able to resume full-time work, and progressively regained my energy and enthusiasm for living, taking on new projects and living life to the full.'

In fact, Jackie completed a Cordon Vert course with the Vegetarian Society, offering the Hay System as her thesis and gaining her Diploma with Distinction. It was as a result of this that Thorsons invited her to write her splendid book *Food Combining for Vegetarians*. She now takes vegetarian cooking classes and lectures on the Hay System – all in addition to a full-time job.

Skin Diseases and Other Allergies

Dr Hay affirmed that he had seen no case of psoriasis
or eczema that did not disappear after a few weeks or a
very few months of separation of incompatible foods –
even though both conditions failed to improve under
the skilled scientific treatment of many prominent skin
specialists.

'Eczema,' wrote Dr Hay, 'is nothing more than
an acid exudate finding exit through the skin, and is
curable by correcting the acid-forming diet to a
neutral or alkaline one, wholly without local application or medication of any kind whatsoever.'

The general belief, however, just as with arthritis, is
that diet is useless for skin diseases. The following case
histories turn this belief upside down:

From a reflexologist:
'One of my patients, a boy of seven, was covered
with psoriasis. He scratched himself until he
bled, his face was scabby, and his scalp was one
complete mass of yellow scab. His body was also
covered. At school children were horrible to him
verbally, and wouldn't play with him in case they
caught it.

'From being a happy child he became very
withdrawn. Within two months of adopting
food combining his scalp and body were
completely clear and he was a lot happier in
himself. A skin specialist he had been attending
was told by his mother what had been done to
resolve the psoriasis, but the specialist insisted

that "no food will make any difference to psoriasis".'

'I would like to thank you for writing *Food Combining for Health*. This book introduced me to the Hay System which has relieved me of eczema, a condition I have had since birth and which always greatly reduced my self–confidence.'

Out of interest – one letter I received from a lady also mentioned her three children, all four of them had allergy problems. She said her son was dyslexic and it was discovered that his dyslexia was attributable to food allergy (in his case milk products, salicylic acid products and three popular food colourings). When he dropped these from his diet his dyslexia improved immensely.

'My allergies hardly cause me any problems since I started the Hay diet. It makes life much more enjoyable.'

'My youngest son, who has always had terrible eczema, has started following the Hay System at last! He is enthralled by the Gordon Grant Loaf and makes it himself! Needless to say, already there is an appreciable improvement in such a short time. He said: "Mum, I wish I'd known about the Hay System before, I needn't have suffered all this time!" I was absolutely speech-less, after all I've only been telling him about it for the last three years or so.'

'The diet was (and still is) a complete success for me. Psoriasis no longer troubles me. I only have the tiniest patch, but most important of all, I feel full of energy and at 57 feel younger than I did 20 years ago.'

'My oldest friend has a daughter who for years has been trying naturopathic remedies for acne, and no success, so I finally persuaded her to try food combining to get rid of her internal toxins and now, three or four weeks into it, the acne has gone and she feels full of life and very well.'

'I am very pleased to say that the improvement of my dermatitis has continued. All the redness has now gone but I still have a facial skin which looks very dry and is still inclined to flakiness. However, I must stress I am very pleased with the progress already made. It is now over five weeks since I last applied steroid cream to my face and I have today condemned to the dustbin all my steroid creams. Just a few months ago, to do this would have been unthinkable.'

'After giving birth to and breast feeding four children in five years, and at the same time passing through a very worrying period for several family members, I entered into a very low state physically, mentally and emotionally. Probably as a result of this I developed what is supposed to be a stress related skin condition – acne rosacea.

'My face and part of my hands were covered in

a dense red rash. Eventually it affected my eyes and I developed cysts all along the eyelids because the tear ducts had become blocked. The surface of the eyes became covered in tiny erosions, and eventually the cornea of one eye was covered by a large ulcer. Over an 18-month period I received long-term antibiotics, antibiotic and cortisone drops for the eyes and cortisone based cream for the face. The condition would start to improve and then worsen. I tried homoeopathic treatments and herbal remedies. I had minor eye surgery to remove some of the larger cysts, and throughout this period attended skin and eye clinics (the eye clinic on a weekly basis).

'One day I was given *Food Combining for Health* by a friend and read in there not only about the Hay diet but also about the benefits of fish oil. I began to take halibut or cod liver oil daily and adopted the principles of food combining. Within three weeks my skin was completely clear and the eye consultant was amazed at the extent of recovery, not only of the skin around the eyelids but of the erosion on the surface of the eye. Within another couple of weeks these had completely healed, leaving only what he described as cortisone damage[!] [perhaps that, too, has gone by now]. I also (very welcome) lost weight and felt a great deal better.

'I should like to add that my daughter at this time was on a very restricted diet which excluded all dairy products, wheat and oats (she is a vegetarian by choice). Even the tiny amount of dairy products or wheat which found its way into her diet caused her to feel nauseous and to have an unpleasant ("cow dung") taste and smell in her mouth. We decided to have a go at the Hay diet (remaining vegetarian) and include all foods in her diet. To her delight she is now able to eat absolutely anything with no side-effects at all. Her hay fever has also greatly diminished. Many thanks.'

'I have just come through a very tough five years of struggle against "total allergy syndrome" (including candida) . . . . I can only tell you that correct combining has been one of the most important factors in my recovery.'

'After reading your book *Food Combining for Health*, my husband and I have enthusiastically followed the diet with much success. Flaky red skin on my husband's face and chest have virtually cleared up, headaches and indigestion are now very rare, and hyperkeratosis on his hands and feet . . . showed unbelievable signs of clearing.'

Three case histories recorded by a retired GP in Scotland:

'In March 1988 the wife of a 51-year-old schoolmaster borrowed my copy of the book. Her husband (whom we shall call Mr X) had suffered from recurring migraine headaches for about 20 years. Blinding headaches recurred several times every week, in some weeks every day. On two occasions recently he had been forced to come home from work at school . . . occasionally his headaches were associated with vomiting; tablets gave some relief if taken in time, and he has tried eliminating from his diet cheese, chocolate and coffee, without effect. His wife, a qualified nurse who had recorded his headaches on a calendar, switched to the food combining system on 25 February 1988; the effect was immediate. No headaches at all were recorded during the whole of March; there was one recurrence in early April when the family were away from home on holiday and could not keep to the food combining rules. To date (June 1988) there has been no recurrence. At the outset of the experiment Mrs X was pretty sceptical about it. Mr X has a family history of migraine and seemed to have resigned himself to the affliction. He is naturally delighted at the transformation in his well-being.'

'Meanwhile, his 18-year-old daughter, Miss X, found that within a few days of starting the new regime, a distressing eczematous rash on the palm of her hands healed completely. She had been using a steroid-containing ointment (Locoid) for symptomatic relief and had been worrying about the effect of this distressing condition on her prospects of employment when she left school. The rash has not recurred.'

'A 56-year-old businessman suffered from blinding headaches associated with "irritable bowel

syndrome" i.e. irregular bowel movements,
abdominal discomfort and sometimes explosive
diarrhoea. Very severe insomnia had plagued him
since 1974 when he had a fairly long spell in
hospital for possible hepatitis. On some nights he
seemed hardly able to sleep at all.

'Four weeks ago he started the food combining
system; his headaches have gone, his insomnia has
greatly improved and his irritable bowel symptoms are much better; he has lost a stone in weight
(dramatic weight loss is a feature of the recorded
effect of the Hay system). Recently on a social
occasion when he could not resist a feast of mince
and potatoes, followed by rice pudding, he
suffered an immediate recurrence of blinding
headache.'

'I've had your book *Food Combining for Health*
for three days and I realize now that wrong
combinations have been my trouble all my life,
but more so in the last few years when – after a
series of medical treatments for MS (which I
haven't got, thank God) – ACTH, dexametha-
sone, tranquillizers, etc. – I developed an "allergic gut". I have been very ill, had to retire, been
to a dozen doctors – even Professor X at Guy's,
and in the end was sent to Mr M in Harley
Street (good job I'm in BUPA). Mr M gives
Potentiated Enzyme Treatment, but although it
is supposed to desensitize against 50 foods, it has
never worked for me for wheat, oats and corn, all
pulses, nuts and seeds, melon, pumpkin and
mango. Now since I've had two days of compati-

ble eating my guts do not blow up to the same extent.'

From Dr X:
'I had ME for 25 years and recently read your book and put it into practice, resulting in a definite increase in energy and well-being. The ME led to candidiasis and numerous food allergies. The Hay diet has been one of the factors which helped me.'

In *Food Combining for Health*, Chapter 3 – 'The Hay System and the Degenerative Diseases' (the section on *allergy*) – the work of Dr John Ott reveals that the *primary* cause of hay fever is a disturbed body chemistry and not the contact with the pollen grains. In other words, the primary cause is the state of the body 'soil' – 'the terrain'!

'Since food combining I don't have hay fever any more, and this was very acute with streaming eyes and nose from breakfast time to after lunch. I was nick-named "The Tissue Lady" because I was never seen without a large box of Kleenex tissues!'

'Two friends both had terrible hay fever. They tell me that they are so much better since going on your diet and will I please say "thank you" to you.'

'I have been using the food combining diet for over a year now and wish I had known about it years ago as I would have saved my daughter years of pain and the agony of hay fever.'

Asthma

One of the commonest chronic allergy diseases today is asthma, the healing of which is stubborn to modern drugs. It is reported as the commonest reason for children going to hospital. For many people it means a lifetime of misery, and it causes 2,000 deaths every year among Britain's three million sufferers.

Now a team of brilliant British scientists has located the gene which causes asthma. According to press reports in 1992, the 'rogue gene' can be hereditary and creates a *'faulty protein'* which can be allergy-causing. The researchers hope to develop a drug which will stop this protein from causing harm, and replace the present drugs and inhalers, some of which may cause serious side-effects.

It appears that asthma victims may have a long wait – about 15 years – before genetic research could lead to a cure. How ironical, therefore, that asthma can be resolved *without drugs, without costly research, and often in the short space of a few weeks – simply by a small change in diet which ensures that the proteins in food are properly digested and do not form this 'faulty protein'*. As discussed in Chapter 2, whether the faulty protein will do harm, or not, may depend largely on the crucial role of diet.

Dr Hay found that this change – to compatible eating – soon allowed his patients to restore to their diet all the health-giving natural foods to which they had formerly been allergic and, impressively, to be able to bury their faces in their former bête noir, whether this was house dust, pollen, animal fur, synthetics or whatever, *without a single sneeze*!

Compatible eating is particularly helpful for asthma. I well remember, over 30 years ago, being sent an elderly asthmatic patient – Cathy – by her doctor, who frankly admitted he could do no more for her. Cathy felt so ill that she was on the point of giving up her job (her sole source of livelihood). She needed no persuasion to adopt food combining principles, and within a few weeks felt so well that she not only retained her job but took on a thrice-weekly evening one as well. Cathy's doctor was delighted (and promptly sent me another of his patients!). I was delighted also – this was my first asthma case. As for Cathy, she remained an enthusiastic devotee of compatible eating for the rest of her life.

From a General Practitioner in Holland:

'Yesterday I saw one of my patients who had a bloated tummy and urticaria when she came to see me. She had these complaints for many years. Now with Hay she is completely cured . . . people of over 50 with a lifetime of tummy aches for the first time becoming free . . . one sufferer from *terrible asthma* now no longer needs her inhaler.'

High Blood-pressure, Cholesterol and Heart Disease

In *Food Combining for Health*, Chapter 4 – 'Butter – Not Margarine' – I revealed how the public is being brainwashed into believing that butter and other animal fats are conducive to heart disease and should be replaced by margarine and vegetable oils. I affirmed that Jean and I do not believe that animal fat is 'the villain of human nutrition'.

Nine years later, Dr John Lockley, in a *Daily Mail* article of 20 April 1993: 'Time to say goodbye to the low fat diet?', explains 'why high cholesterol food may not be the villain in the heart attack story'. His explanation is too long and too complicated to discuss here, but his personal opinion in the penultimate paragraph is worth recording: 'Personally, I think that by the turn of the century we will look back at "the great cholesterol myth" and wonder how we could have been so blind as to miss the truth for so long.*'

During the past decade there have been many studies which question the theory that a switch from

* Since this section was written, research by Melbourne scientists at the Alfred and Baker Unit has revealed that hundreds of thousands of Australians may be able to stop the drugs – ACE inhibitors prescribed to be taken by patients for life in order to keep blood pressure down. According to Steve Dow, medical reporter of The Age, this research could force a rethink on drug use and lead to fundamental changes in medical thinking; it has shown that these ACE inhibitors can be replaced with 'flexible exercise and good diet'! The findings of the Melbourne scientists will be presented to a meeting of the European Society of Hypertension in Milan in June 1995 (The Age, 7 April 1995).

saturated to polyunsaturated fat prevents coronary thrombosis. One study in particular, of great interest, was published in *The Lancet*, 16 November 1985: 'Diet and Risk Factors for Coronary Heart Disease in Asians in North West London', by P. M. McKeigue and co-workers. Moreover, according to Peter Elwood writing in *Yorkshire Medicine*, 1991: 'The absence of clear evidence of a reduction in mortality from trials of dietary fat reduction indicates the need for fresh thinking on the value of dietary fat reduction . . . this conclusion has been reached by a number of authors.'

The findings of a more recent 10-year study at Harvard Medical School, published in *The Lancet* in March 1993, strongly support the conclusions of many authorities today – that the recommended switch from saturated animal fats to much-lauded polyunsaturated vegetable fats has not produced the anticipated benefits and, instead, is actually contributing to the occurrence of coronary heart disease.Coronary disease is now the biggest cause of death in Britain, and is linked to unhealthy eating and lack of exercise. Using a new technique that detects the first signs of the fatal illness in young people, doctors at Great Ormond Street Hospital, London, made the shattering discovery in 1994 of *heart disease in children under 10 years of age*! This technique, however, is still in the development stage, and it may be some time before a screening test to pick up young heart attack candidates will be routinely available.

That harm can result from a low fat diet is suggested by the two following letters:

'I found that I was not taking enough fat in my diet to absorb the calcium and vitamins A and D, and consequently I was suffering from pains in my eyes and mucous colitis, gnawing indigestion and backache on waking in the morning. Although I was taking vitamin tablets they were not being absorbed. I have now gone back to a full-cream milk and have a little fat in my diet, and I have found that this has solved my problems – no backache, no colitis.'

'Hello again. As promised I am writing to report the result of using the "diet" – I should say fantastic diet. Well, life has taken on new meaning, and although I do still suffer from rhinitis at times, I would say that it is 80 per cent better, and no doubt it will get better still. I have also lost half a stone . . . . I make the Grant Loaf and it is wonderful. I have discovered that the margarine I was using was one of the causes of the allergy. I now use butter and am much better. I could hardly believe the difference.'

To conclude this chapter I would like to quote the following example, illustrating how food combining can assail various disorders in one fell swoop, completely enhancing family life for the better.

Food Combining Changed Our Lives

The August 1993 issue of *Here's Health* contained a remarkable story of an English family in Spain – mother, father and two young daughters – and their battle against constant ill health, chronic asthma, arthritis, allergies, weight problems, depression, lethargy and juvenile behavioural aberrations of surliness and aggression.

The article, written by Janette, the mother, related how 'food combining changed our lives' (to quote its caption in huge red capitals). Life was a disaster, and all Janette could think of was whether or not they all had enough drugs (Becotide, Ventolin, etc.) to get everybody through the day. As well as these conventional drugs, wrote Janette, 'they took herbal remedies, homoeopathic concoctions and every piece of advice from logical and sensible to the weird and sometimes ludicrous. Nothing worked. We remained constantly ill, lethargic and generally miserable. And we suffered bouts of distressing allergic reactions about which it seemed we could do nothing.'

Then, when Janette was at her lowest ebb (August 1992), 'crying hysterically', someone handed her a copy of *Food Combining for Health*. 'I swear it changed our lives . . . . The results have been staggering. My allergies have all but disappeared . . . . I sleep well . . . . The arthritis is barely a twinge on damp mornings . . . . I feel relaxed and more able to cope . . . . Howard's asthma disappeared almost overnight, along with the attendant depression which left him dragging himself along for months . . . . Within days Janicka's breathing problems disappeared . . . the detested flab fell away to reveal enviable sleekness she could not previously achieve. She is so delighted with her new figure that nothing would persuade her to go back to our old ways!'

About her other daughter, Charis, Janette wrote:

'Her behaviour worsened for a couple of weeks, but slowly she came round. By March this year [1993] she was a different child. Her eczema cleared up by degrees until Christmas when she wore short sleeves at a party without feeling self-conscious. She's always smiling now, and is a pleasure to live with . . . . If all this sounds too good to be true, there's more! The most phenomenal result of our new diet has been in the change of energy levels. No more lethargy, apathy or depression. Jobs get well done and with smiling enthusiasm and I no longer have to drag everyone out of bed in the mornings, they're up and about often before I am, laughing and chattering about their plans for the day.

'Howard has started to build a terrace at the rear of the house. Every evening he works on it cheerfully and with seemingly endless energy after a long day at work – he is a horticulturist. Before the Hay diet this would have been impossible. He would never have had the energy to do the work, even if he hadn't been allergic to the building materials.

'Both children have taken up action sports which they could not do before. They can sniff at flowers and tree blossoms without collapsing in a wheezing heap. They have roller boots and bicycles, and it is a marvellous thing to watch the people I love most in the world in their new-found health. All this happiness has come in just 10 months, thanks to a small book and the quiet foresight of someone who understands the value of Dr Hay's work. We are once again a family since we tossed away the old anxieties along with boxloads of medication . . . .'

No wonder Janette claimed that food combining changed the lives of her family!

The authors of *Food Combining for Health* feel immensely rewarded that devotees of the Hay lifestyle find that they have not only resolved or ameliorated long-standing health problems – in many cases miraculously – but also have never felt so well.

4

Unexpected Benefits

Health and vitality are our divine birthright; we were created to be well. There is an underlying pattern of perfection awaiting expression within every cell and atom of the body. By following Hay rules you can release this perfection in many astonishing ways. This can happen in a number of ways that are unexpected and mainly unheard of, as the following accounts confirm.

Morning Sickness Banished

It is not generally known, for instance, that observing Hay rules can prevent 'morning sickness'. What a tremendous boon this knowledge could be for thousands of pregnant women who suffer from it. In the Thalidomide era this knowledge could have prevented the birth of thousands of tragically deformed babies whose mothers were prescribed Thalidomide for morning sickness and sleeplessness.

In *The Book of Earthly Delights* by Abbie Heathcote and Neil Douglas[1], Neil recounts how his wife,

Vivienne, was suffering so badly with morning sickness that she decided to try the Hay diet. All their friends 'rubbished' the diet, but finally their morning sickness forced the sceptics to try it out. Vivienne's mother, a nurse, thought the diet was a lot of nonsense, but Vivienne had no morning sickness as long as she stuck rigidly to the rules. If she did have a bout of sickness, her husband would ask her what she had eaten; and they could always track down the cause to some little thing that she had eaten absent-mindedly or without realizing it was against the rules. 'One day she was vomiting and was sure that she had eaten nothing wrong. Then she remembered that she had eaten half a plum, plucked from the tree as she walked in the garden. Dr Hay ruled out plums on the grounds that they contain an indigestible acid, which the body finds very hard to eliminate. Another bout was caused by eating half a biscuit in the wrong combination, too soon before or after she had eaten protein or acid fruit.'

Neil Douglas also recounts how a scientist friend believed that the Hay diet, scientifically, was a lot of nonsense. This friend and his wife wanted a big family, but his wife's nausea and vomiting were so bad that she had gone to many doctors, ending up at specialists in Collins Street – the Melbourne equivalent of Harley Street – who were also unable to help. These friends wrote to Neil and his wife, saying that they had a friend who had a very serious morning sickness problem, and they wanted to tell her about the Hay diet as she had tried everything else. The 'friend', however, turned out to be the scientist's wife, who admitted later that she wanted to try the diet herself, in desperation, after the specialists had failed to help her. *The Hay diet worked immediately!*

(Incidentally, if exhausted nursing mothers who have crying and colicky babies would try combining their foods according to Hay principles, they may be astonished at the pacifying effect.)

Alcohol Addiction Conquered

In a remarkable letter recently received, the writer relates how, two years ago, she came out of an Addiction Treatment Centre after nine weeks of intensive therapy, but was *very* ill:

'I had stomach ulcers, gout, Reynaud's Disease, epileptic seizures, cervical spondylosis and, worst of all, peripheral neuritis – a very painful debilitating condition which had also seriously affected my brain.

'Just three weeks following Hay, and I no longer needed drugs for the ulcers or the gout – and these conditions have not returned. Within a few months I stopped taking phenytoin and have had no recurrence of epileptic attack. The other conditions are long-standing, having taken years to develop – and my GP told me they would take years to heal. She was very enthusiastic when I told her I was following Dr Hay's system, and advised me to continue – adding that she, herself, had been a devotee for many years.

'You should see me now! I am like a new person – in mind, body and spirit. Despite many shattering events that have occurred in my life during the past two years, I remain fit, slim and "together" – able to cope. I can honestly say, with grateful thanks, that Dr Hay's system, and your own advice, has achieved this "Lazarus-like" rebirth.

'I just had to tell you what the Hay System has done for me!'

I have met the young woman who wrote this letter and was greatly impressed with her appearance and philosophy of life. She often stays with relatives who do a great deal of drinking, but her self-discipline is remarkable; for over three and a half years not one drop of alcohol has passed her lips and she feels no need or craving for it any more.

Another outstanding letter about addiction – in this case to chocolate – was recorded in a recent edition of *Food Combining for Health*, and is worth recording here. The writer had been ill for over 20 years, was overweight, and in desperation had followed 'endless diets' with limited success. She had also been to an allergy clinic which had helped with depression and 'irritable bowels'. She had also been going to therapy sessions run by her GP to try to come to terms with the eating habits and chocolate addiction which were ruining her life:

'Now after following your advice I am delighted to find that my chocolate addiction has gone. Since I started to follow your ways, I have not eaten any at all, and I was previously trying to cut down on three Mars bars a day! I have not even wanted to eat chocolate, which is even more miraculous, as I was really hooked, and suffered the most trying withdrawal symptoms when I gave it up before. My headaches have gone, and the joint pains and stiffness which were making me feel like an old woman (I am nearly 40) have disappeared. As a bonus I have lost 2 lb. in weight this week, and I have been eating good amounts of food at each meal.'

Hiatus Hernia Resolved

Hiatus hernia is a most trying and unpleasant complaint. As one correspondent wrote: 'My daughter has a hereditary hiatus hernia – the stomach doesn't close properly and food is coming up to her mouth all the time (wear and tear on her teeth – not very pleasant smell).'

In *The Saccharine Disease*, Surgeon Capt. T. L. Cleave's famous book[2], there is a description on page 176 of the mechanism involved in hiatus hernia: '. . . just as the oesophageal sphincter contracts strongly in a fast emptying time, so it will relax in a sluggish one. And it is this relaxation that the author submits allows the oesophageal reflux ("acid eructation" and "heartburn") that initiates, and is always the hallmark of hiatus hernia.'

In other words, if the emptying of the stomach is sluggish, the 'oesophageal sphincter' (OS) relaxes, and this prevents the stomach from closing. Then there are unpleasant acid eructations and heartburn. If the emptying of the stomach is fast, the OS contracts properly and there is no acid eructation or heartburn.

Both Pavlov[3] and Dr Lionel Picton[4] (*see Chapter 2*) revealed by their own research on digestion that incompatible mixtures of food greatly slow down the emptying time of the stomach. This can cause the OS to relax – hence the eructations. Here is yet more evidence – and vindication – of the wisdom and benefits of Dr Hay's starch/protein rule.

'We are very recent converts to the Hay diet. My husband was recommended to try it for his hiatus hernia. He has had tummy ache for a number of years – he is 36. From being very poorly only a few weeks ago, he now suffers no tummy ache at all!'

'Your book has really been a boon. I have had all sorts of illnesses throughout my life, but this unruly stomach has been an awful bane. And how lovely to be able to sleep at night.'

'My daughter's mother-in-law has experienced great relief from hiatus hernia since I introduced her to food combining some 18 months ago.'

'I have been suffering from chronic flatulence for many years, in fact it had made my life a misery – not being able to get rid of it, consequently being robbed of sleep, not knowing a good night's sleep in all that time. I must mention I was diagnosed as having a hiatus hernia and diverticulitis, and being treated medically for these conditions with every proprietary brand of medicine in turn – all to no avail. I bought *Food Combining for Health* but it seemed very formidable. I stuck to it for about a month and gave up in despair – it didn't work straightaway as some of the people claimed in the book. I realize now I wasn't being strict enough, e.g. still having biscuits with morning coffee and afternoon tea, etc. I didn't see how it was possible to do without following the habit of a lifetime. (I am now 58).

'I was suffering so much, also with terrible heartburn, that I started once more with more determination. I have now been food combining for about 12 months and am pleased to say there is a very real improvement. I'd like to add that I can now eat lettuce, cucumber, onions and bananas without any trouble – food items I'd not had for years because of the awful indigestion they gave me.'

'In 1971 I was diagnosed as having hiatus hernia and was prescribed medication to combat the effects of this. As time went by I found it necessary to increase the frequency of medi-cation. To add to this problem, in 1982 and 1984 I suffered coronaries and was left with angina and ischaemic heart disease. Medication for this created gout pains, and to combat these I now take further medication. Despite this I often have pain from the gout.

'In 1992 I decided to give food combining a try, and within a few months the hiatus hernia was giving less trouble and I was able to level out the medication to a realistic figure. Pain in my leg is less frequent and less intense; however, the medication must continue – the surgery I attend looks after me very well and I am examined frequently.

'Recently I had a check for cholesterol and blood-pressure, and a urine test. My blood-pressure was perfect, I was informed, and there were no problems with the water test. The cholesterol level was 4:1 and this was on a full-fat diet, i.e. butter, all-fat milk, etc.

'I know this plan works for me, and I firmly believe it is because I do not cheat. I confess it takes quite a lot of resolve not to cheat. But that is a small price to pay for the amount of relief I now enjoy. Give it a go – the only thing you can lose is the pain!

'In addition, I am now eating foods that I have not been able to eat for years – cucumber, pickles (home-made), onions in cooking, cream, even garlic, all of which would bring about severe eructation from the hiatus hernia, also angina pains.'

Groin Hernia Resolved

Repair for groin hernia is one of the most common operations – there are about 80 thousand hernia repairs per year. In 1988 this was estimated to have cost the NHS £344 million, and correcting those repairs which failed – according to a press report in April 1993 – could cost the NHS around £5 million per year. Surgery, however, is medically acknowledged to be the only way to repair a groin hernia. The following account of a groin hernia, resolved *without surgery* after about nine months of food combining, is therefore of special interest. It turned out to be quite a saga!

'Nearly three years ago I suffered an accidental fall, causing a strain/sprain in the lower part of my back, resulting in loss of work and severe pain for the following five to six weeks. There was also a pain, and swelling in the shape of an egg, in my left groin.

'As my back was improving and groin pain was not, my doctor gave me what I believe to be a very thorough and completely unhurried examination – so thorough in fact that he re-checked almost the whole of the examination process. His opinion was a "Direct" hernia in the groin. He believed I needed surgery and arranged for me to see a specialist.

'I called at the local Reference Library and looked up a medical dictionary on hernias. From my understanding of this reference work, it appeared the symptoms and the pains I was suffering seemed to correspond to what I was reading. Official and unofficial enquiries of medical opinion seemed to indicate quite firmly that there was no alternative to surgery.

'I mentioned the events to you at the time and I vividly recall your advice: "Don't hurry to get surgery and do tighten up on the food combining rules." Tightening up on food combining rules was virtually impossible – I carried them out to the letter anyway!

'After the initial three months or so when the pain was quite intense, the swelling and the pain gradually subsided, so that when I did see the specialist some eight to nine months after the accident, there were no indications whatsoever. I felt nothing and there was no swelling.

'After my examination, the specialist announced, quite annoyed I thought, that I did not have a hernia. He somewhat grudgingly muttered something about a muscle strain, and that I would not be needing surgery. In the adjoining room, I heard what must have been the dictation of a letter back to my GP. I did not exactly hear what was said, but the tone was unmistakable.

'I feel genuinely sorry for my GP, a very pleasant man; it must have been very humiliating for him – after his very careful examination and positive diagnosis – to virtually be forced to admit to a wrong diagnosis; especially as a groin hernia diagnosis was one of those a doctor was least likely to make a mistake over.

'I should have had an examination by the specialist a week or so after the diagnosis; I would then have known exactly what the position is. As it happens we will never know.'

Anti-ageing Benefits –
Feeling and Looking Younger

There is now an anti-ageing, anti-wrinkling pill on the market – 'the first internal cosmetic', according to its distributors – *but it costs nearly £1 per day!*

According to press reports in 1993, some people found this pill 'absolutely wonderful'. Other people found it disappointing, but some skin specialists using it in their clinics found it 'spectacular'. Most people found that the biggest skin changes were improved skin textures, diminishing pore size, and more even colour, with a healthy glow.

Countless women have experienced similar anti-ageing effects on a food combining diet, but *at no cost whatsoever*. It worked even when accompanied by a skin disease, as in the case of Mary Anne Shearer. Her story, told in 1989 in *The Star* South Africa by Caroline Hurry, is particularly dramatic. For two years she had been sneezing solidly, and for two years relentless attacks of dermatitis, which failed to respond to cortisone treatment, had cracked her skin open. Moreover, she constantly suffered from colds, 'flu and sinus attacks. She felt desperate and depressed; neither doctor nor homoeopath could help her. *But food combining worked immediately.* The day she started the diet her sneezing stopped and a week later her dermatitis disappeared. Within two months she lost 12 kg to reach her ideal weight. Her energy level shot up and she 'felt fantastic'. 'Today, Mrs Shearer's complexion glows like peaches and cream, and she exudes the energy of a racehorse at the starter gate. Her secret? Nothing more than correct food combining.'

Greatly Increased Energy and Feeling Much Younger

Energy is the theme song in many letters from food combining enthusiasts: How much more energy they have and how much younger they feel, as related in the previous chapter:

'It is years since I felt so well and happy – now at 60, I feel 10 years younger than I did at 50.'

'I feel full of energy and at 57 feel younger than I did 20 years ago.'

'For three months I avoided eating starch and protein at the same meal and very soon I felt much younger and fitter and more energetic.'

'I am thrilled to be feeling so well and so young again.'

The Hay System is indeed a most effective anti-ageing diet!

Recovery Without Drugs from Viral and Fungal Infections

In her most helpful and splendidly researched book, *The Ordinary Person's Guide to 'Extraordinary Health'*[5] Jillie Collings writes:

'In the last ten to twenty years we have seen an alarming increase in the severity of the effects of certain viruses and fungi on general health, such as Coxsackie, Zoster varicella and Epstein-Barr viruses, which can feature in ME and in Candida albicans, the yeast-like organism that can become, under certain circumstances, fungal in nature, penetrate the wall of the gut and therefore pour toxins into the bloodstream.'

Jillie Collings points out that these, 'together with the increasing incidence of allergies, PMT and infections like ME, resistant strains of VD, infectious hepatitis, and AIDS, are challenging health authorities and their resources to the extreme.'

She also points out that many of the drugs prescribed to fight these conditions are further polluting our insides, which are already subjected to the pollution of our environment in food, air, water and earth.

The following extracts from two letters suggest that the Hay System principles can effect recovery from viral and fungal infections in a way which orthodox medicines in many cases cannot:

'I have had labyrinthitis followed by post viral fatigue syndrome – off work for four months – doctors no help but am now back on my feet because of – you've guessed it – THE HAY DIET. I am so grateful.'

'In 1980 – I was struck down with a severe illness which the doctor and specialist informed me was muscular myasthenia, an extreme form of muscle debility caused by a virus – I'm almost on my way to full recovery due to the fact that I was a very active and fit sportswoman before the illness struck. Also I firmly believe it is because I'm on the "Hay Diet", or should I say Hay way of life!

'Before my illness I was 10 stone 10 lb. at 5 ft. 7½in. tall. During the illness I accumulated a lot of weight due to immobility. I went up to 12 stone 8 lb. plus. Since I started the "Hay" way of life, I'm now 10 stone 7 lb. and still losing about 2 lb. per week. I never feel hungry, or crave sweet things. I eat as much as I want, bearing always in mind *never* to mix foods that fight. I have more energy, am more mentally alert, my skin and hair is quite unbelievable, and the fungus which covered my body is now gone, my stress and muscular incontinence has also gone. I'm now able to sleep, feel a lot calmer in myself. I found it hard to believe that a clean way of eating could change my whole life, but the proof of the pudding is certainly in the "eating".

'I look to each meal with great excitement and

no longer drink tea or coffee; that was the hardest to give up, as I *do*, or did, enjoy my cups of tea and coffee. However, I do drink herbal tea or just fresh lemon and water, and I don't have heavy shopping bills or baskets, and spend less time shopping.

'I want to thank you for this wonderful way of life. I shall keep you informed regarding my health and weight.'

Possible Protection Against HIV

In many cases the drugs prescribed for fungal and virus infections become more lethal than the diseases. This fact is strikingly revealed in the title of an article in *The International Journal of Alternative and Complementary Medicine*, April 1993, by Dr G. Orth of Leutkirch, Germany: 'Cause of death – AIDS therapy'.

Research which Dr Orth carried out with the help of a well-known industrial foundation led to astonishing results. Very briefly, he found that AIDS is not a uniform infectious disease (it can consist of many diseases) but has to do with a systemic condition of the whole body, 'and only conditionally has anything to do with the HI virus.' Dr Orth established that in every case that came to his knowledge, 'the patient had already been immune-suppressed by drugs or antibiotics or some other heavy immune suppressant'; that the HI virus seems to creep in after an earlier immune suppression and, moreover, that this suppression is augmented by the clinical treatment at present given to AIDS patients, as every medicine used in AIDS is immune suppressive. In every case he knew, the orthodox therapy, with drugs and antibiotics led to death.*

Of special interest to food combiners is the fact, according to Dr Orth, that a patient with full-blown AIDS always has a low pH. This low pH of the body fluids appears to be the only milieu in which the virus can live. 'If this milieu [*terrain*], is changed,' writes Dr Orth, 'the HI virus is no longer capable of living. It is not the virus that may be allowed to determine the terrain but the patient.'

Once again, nutrition would seem to be the whole crux of the matter. Apart from a number of different therapies (such as antiviral herbs and correcting harmful lifestyles) Dr Orth particularly recommends *an alteration of the diet to alkaline-producing foods* and states that it is important that the fruit and vegetable intake should be increased to 75 per cent of the total, and that 25 per cent should be raw. The acid-producing foods (meat, cheese, eggs, and so on) should be reduced to about 20 per cent, he says.

Pure Hay System!

As well as being largely alkaline-forming, such a diet is immune system supportive. According to Dr Orth it is also the main requisite for combating a fungal infection: 'Since fungi live in an acidic medium,

---

*In April 1993, AZT – hailed as a wonder drug – was revealed to be useless in delaying the onset of AIDS. Because of the toxicity for immune cells, it was pronounced 'AIDS by prescription' by Peter Duesbery, world authority on viruses and Professor of Molecular Biology, University of California, Berkeley.

the source of nutriment plays a key role. The food-stuffs must be alkaline-producing.'

Dr Orth's article is remarkable vindication of Dr Hay's principles, especially his concept that the secret of optimum health and resistance to disease lies in the correct alkalinity of the body, the alkaline/acid balance – *In other words, an effective immune system.*

Dr Walb and The Hay System

Dr Orth's obvious familiarity with Hay principles strongly suggests that he was acquainted with the works and Hay writings of a contemporary German physician, Dr Walb.

In *The Superfoods Diet Book*[6] (full of excellent food combining recipes), Michael Van Straten and Barbara Griggs relate how, in 1939, a young German doctor chanced on Dr Hay's diet, and how he tried it on a nine-year-old boy, 'who had been suffering pain from an advanced kidney disease for which conventional medicine could offer no cure. To his amazement, Dr Hay's regime brought an almost immediate improvement, and eventually, a cure.'

At the clinic he set up in Ohm after the war, Dr Walb with his wife and partner, Dr Ilse Walb, adopted the Hay regime as standard treatment for a long list of diseases, 'that were strikingly alleviated and often completely cured by this diet alone.'

The book this husband and wife team wrote, *Die Haysche Trennskost*, went to 39 editions and became a bestseller in Germany from the late 1950s. In Italy it ran through 20 printings in just four years.

Such success with the Hay System is now wide-spread; it is a 'normalising' diet. The 'normal', (not to be confused with 'the average'), means perfect functioning of every cell and atom of our 'fearfully and wonderfully made bodies'.

Colitis

This letter was published in *Grace* magazine, Spring 1992:

'I lost and regained my health last year. From mid-April I suffered constant, unremitting diarrhoea. I tried all supplements, vitamins and homoeopathic remedies; gradually eliminating everything from my diet that seemed to make it worse; finally I succumbed to the medical profession and had all the tests. Colitis was diagnosed and treatment by cortisone and sulphonamides was prescribed.

'At first this treatment worked like a miracle – but with side-effects and joint pains, dizziness on rising, feverish nightmares. In the end, though, the colitis gradually overcame the medicine and I was reduced to eating cheese and bread, cereal and milk and mashed potatoes. I hit an all-time low one Sunday with nausea and vomiting, feeling terrible even lying down.

'Then, I read about the Hay Diet. What had I to lose? The effects were instantaneous! No diarrhoea, no vomiting, no pain or discomfort – and with no medication! It was an end to joint

pains and nightmares. Two days later I looked
in the mirror and thought: Hi! I know you. You
used to live here – welcome back!

'I now feel absolutely wonderful, better than
for years, and the diet is so simple and full of
good things. Devotees will recognize that by
reducing to bread/cheese, cereal/milk, etc., I
was making myself sicker by the day – the principle being that protein and starch don't mix if
taken at the same meal.'

Women's Health?

Sadly, I have heard from no Hay devotees that problems which frequently beset the gentler sex – PMT,
troublesome menopause, cellulite, painful periods –
are helped or prevented on a well-established Hay
lifestyle. I can only confirm that for me all these conditions were completely non-existent. A friend states
from her own experience that cellulite disappeared
without the use of special creams or exercises, simply
noticing that it was no longer a problem some nine
months from commencing to 'Hay'.

By a strange coincidence, however, the very
day after the foregoing paragraph was written, the
following letter was in my morning post. It was from
a woman who had suffered terrible period pains
for many years. She also had irritable bowel syndrome, brought on, she was told, by 20 years of
anti-depressants, and painkillers for her sciatica. She
wrote:

'I have now been food combining for five weeks. I am pleased to find that my back has not given me any noticeable pain for a fortnight, and I am in the middle of a heavy period but having no pain. The pain is usually so terrible that painkillers are useless and I end up rolling on the floor! I have lost 5 lb., and that constant craving for food I have had all my life is nearly gone. I can go four hours without eating anything but a small hand-ful of sunflower seeds.

'I used to feel terribly ill in the afternoons and had to go to bed for an hour. I still rest, because I am tired (I am an insomniac), but I no longer feel ill. I am so grateful.'

The writer of the following letter had nearly every-thing wrong with her except housemaid's knee! It was addressed to me c/o The Food Programme, Radio 4, and was prompted by the 'Food Combining' broad-cast on 18 June 1993, for which I was interviewed:

'I would like to thank you for changing my life so dramatically. Three years ago at the age of 48, I was getting fed up with having cystitis repeat-edly, migraines monthly, and almost permanent upset stomach, tennis elbow and fatigue and although not really over-weight, but thick around my waist and feeling I could be slimmer, I bought your book [*Food Combining for Health*] and have *never* looked back. All these symptoms have disappeared, my weight is constant at 9½ stones and my waist is smaller and my bosom bigger!!! Also the best present was being able to drink red wine without having a hangover, and being able to drink more.'

Strangely, the following remarkable letter (dated 24 February 1995) was also prompted by a broadcast of The Food Programme on Radio 4, and again one in which I had taken part. It was from 'a just-post-menopausal woman (54)', as she described herself, and she said she wrote 'as a brand-new convert to Dr Hay's way of living.' It was addressed to Derek Cooper, who kindly gave me permission to quote it, as also did the writer herself:

'After Christmas, as many of us do, I felt fat, frowsty and fed-up with my increasingly indulgent and unsuitable diet. I had also been anxious for some time about the unmistakable signs of rheumatic problems – creaky knees, lumpy finger-joints, aches and stiffness after exercise etc. I bought a book on food combining, and, thinking it would at any rate shift some of my surplus pounds, I went shopping for fruit, a yoghourt-maker, lots of vegetables and began.

'At the risk of sounding like a testimonial, I have to report results so startling that I can hardly believe them myself.

'First, without ever feeling hungry I have lost ten pounds, and now have once more the figure I thought had gone with my child-bearing years. Second, what I'm eating is so good that I can't wait for the next meal. Thirdly, my joints feel as though they've been oiled, and my finger lumps are diminishing.

'In addition to this I have enormous new energy and sense of optimism, and I sleep and concentrate better. My food bills have dropped and I've never cooked food which is quicker or simpler to prepare.

'This isn't a slimming diet, and I shan't revert because I prefer it. And contrary to what people sometimes suggest, it's not difficult to reconcile with eating out or feeding a family. In fact, as two of my women friends will testify, you can put your man on the Hay diet without him knowing!

'The Hay attitude to low-fat, so called 'healthy', products has excellent consequences. For example, in today's food fad world, it's such a relief to mind and taste buds to be told that with a properly-balanced mainly alkaline diet, there's nothing wrong with moderate amounts of good unsalted butter. So don't buy additive-laden spreads in the belief that you're doing yourself good.

'Please devote some more airtime to this way of eating – it's such a simple trick with so many benefits.'

Relief from Stressful Side-effects After a Cancer Operation and Possible Prevention of Cancer

According to the World Cancer Research Fund Newsletter, Spring 1993, many scientists now estimate that over a third of cancer deaths may be prevented through dietary means.

That food combining principles may be of particular value in such prevention is suggested by a letter received from a famous Dutch physician who uses food combining in his practice, Hans Moolenburgh: 'I believe that in a time of vast environmental pollution the diet helps in quicker detoxification through better elimination.' He suggests that a survey should be done amongst people who really keep to the diet to find out if they have less cancer than a 'normal' eating population. 'It is my opinion,' he writes, 'that you would find some astonishing results and the only thing to be done is to give the suggestion a try.'

As well as a possible prevention of cancer, it would appear that food combining can be of invaluable help in preventing or ameliorating painful and stressful side-effects after a cancer operation. This fact came to light in a letter from a woman who endured four years of constant abdominal pain and anxiety after her cancer operation. She wrote:

'I was feeling so ill by June this year with the pain, faintness, lack of energy, lack of co-ordination (I love to play the piano and it is

becoming so frustrating) and a feeling of not
being able to cope, that I was actually devising
possible "foolproof" methods of suicide! Because
life seemed only to be full of worry and pain,
with no help or hope offered by those who were
supposed to be helping me.

'On adopting food combining, and experiencing the upswing of well-being, I knew that I was
onto something important. I *was* sceptical, but
now, since feeling so much better, I see it all
makes sense. I have found that eminent doctors –
my doctor is said to be one of the best in the
country (NHS) – still don't seem to be aware of
the faults of modern "normal diet". I was very
angry that I had suffered four years of pain and
anxiety, and that my consultant and GP *never
once* pointed in the direction of any book on diet.
I really think they should have made it their business to be aware of these things and not just leave
the poor patients to their own devices.'

It would appear that food combining can indeed
ameliorate the painful, stressful, life-threatening side-
effects after a cancer operation. In her book, *The Food
Combining Diet* (Thorsons, 1993), Kathryn Marsden
describes how food combining finally restored her
husband to health after *two* major cancer operations –
one for the complete removal of his stomach, and the
second 'which divorced him from his spleen'. The
side-effects were appallingly painful and no-one
thought he would live. Kathryn writes that she and her
husband were shown much kindness and sympathy,
but there was 'a dearth of practical help' from the

medical experts and dieticians etc. (Just as was the experience of the writer of the foregoing letter).

It was thanks to Kathryn's quite remarkable perseverance in researching all life-saving aspects of nutritional therapies and to her adoption of food combining, which finally saved her husband's life. And he is still well. She is to be heartily congratulated on an outstanding achievement.

Recovery from Prostate Trouble

Letter to the Director of the Prostate Help Association:

'I'm aged 55 years and, until last September, had for some seven or eight years lived with all the symptoms mentioned in the leaflet you enclosed. That apart, I was (and still am) in very good health and judged that the condition was not sufficiently serious to warrant bothering my GP on that matter alone. About nine months ago I visited my GP at my wife's behest concerning a couple of warts on my leg. At that visit I made passing mention of "the symptoms" and, on examination, an enlarged prostate was diagnosed. The GP referred me to a specialist who, following the usual tests, confirmed the GP's diagnosis.

'The specialist didn't view my problem as sufficiently advanced to warrant an operation, but did suggest tablets (which would have to be taken for the rest of my life) to alleviate the symptoms. I can't recall that he named the tablets, and I didn't ask, although I did ask what the side-effects would be. He said possibly dryness of the mouth and a tendency for drowsiness. I said I'd think about it.

'My story now goes back to Easter 1991 when we met a Scottish couple on holiday in Madeira who were staying in the same hotel as us. Her name was Doris Grant, who'd co-written with Jean Joice a book called *Food Combining for Health* which had just been reprinted. At that time Mrs Grant was aged 86 and her husband 89. Both gave the appearance of people 20 years younger – particularly Mr Grant who was quite remarkable for a man of his age. On our return from holiday I happened to see the book in Smiths and, out of interest, bought it. In simple terms, the book advocates not mixing in the same meal certain combinations of food, such as carbohydrates with protein and other combinations claimed to have a deleterious effect on one's health. The book doesn't claim cures, but rather that the system allows natural inbuilt healing powers of the body to reign; from arthritis to allergies and gall stones to chronic migraine. Having read this book, I put it to one side.

'Coming back to more recent times, I got to thinking about what the specialist had to say. In no way did I fancy being on a regime of tablets for the rest of my life, particularly with the possibility of side-effects as described. I took the view that treating the symptoms – which is all that the tablets would do – wasn't the answer. I wanted to address the *cause* of the symptoms. It was at this point I asked my wife to arrange my meals to adhere to that advanced by Doris Grant in her book.

'I can't begin to understand how combining food in a certain way can have any particular nutritional merit or facilitate better the body's natural healing. All I can say is that within days of changing the composition of my meals substantially along the lines (I won't pretend not to having the occasional lapse now and then) suggested in the book, the symptoms of the diagnosed swollen prostate diminished. I now seldom need to visit the lavatory during the night. As this occurred without any medication or other treatment, I can only conclude that my prostate has receded to something approaching its normal size. Other evident side-effects are the complete loss of a quite sharp low back pain which I'd lived with for many years since quite a young man and had always put down to back strain, common (so I'd been told) in tall people, and some weight loss, albeit that I didn't have any particular weight problem. Correct food combining is not a diet for losing weight as such, and as most of us are heavier than we should be, weight loss is a natural consequence. The quantity of my food intake has not altered – I still eat as much as I want. This includes breakfast, three course lunch and evening meal; and I'm not averse to pre-bedtime supper on the not infrequent occasion. I conclude that if a person were under weight, the tendency would be to become heavier from correct food combining.

'I'm not seeking to advocate food combining as a solution – I'm not qualified to do so. I'd be loath to support any theory which I can't myself comprehend. All I can do is re-tell what happened to me. I accept that other coincident factors could have come into play at the time I addressed the issue of food combining last September, but I can't think of any. I suppose I could revert to random food mixing in my meals to prove a point by seeing if my old problems re-emerge, but frankly I've become too used to not tripping my toe-stubbing 3 a.m. route to the lavatory each morning, to risk it!

'I present my experience for others to note and comment.'

Happiness

Health and happiness usually go together. They certainly appear to do so judging from the expression of new-found happiness in so many of the letters received from successful food combiners.

Happiness, in itself, is health-giving. Unhappiness, on the other hand, can be health-destroying. As I have written elsewhere, all the negative emotions such as fear, jealousy, hatred, temper, criticism and sadness, destroy health by setting free – creating – poisonous acids in the system and lowering the precious alkaline reserve of the body. This sets up a vicious circle because acidity appears to irritate the cells of the nervous system, making people super-critical, truculent, bad-tempered and quarrelsome. This, in turn, creates more tension and results in still more acidity.

'The greatest cause of disease,' claimed Joe Nichols, distinguished American doctor and President of Natural Food Associates, 'even greater than faulty nutrition, is without doubt emotional . . . . I know a man who has gout. He gets along very well until he gets mad; then he has to go to hospital.' The late Sir Heneage Ogilvie, consultant surgeon at Guy's Hospital, shared this view. In a remarkable paper in *The Lancet*, July 1957, such as had never before been published in a medical journal, he suggested that disaster, bereavement or unhappiness can 'trigger off' latent cancer, and on the other hand, that the happy man is captain of his cells and master of his fate, and thereby immune from certain diseases.

Dr Hay was well aware of these facts and never forgot to stress the importance of positive thinking to health. This may well explain the benefit of new-found, unexpected happiness experienced by successful devotees of the Hay System.

5

Matters of Consequence

Quite apart from the known dangers of suspect additives in the food we eat, of health-destroying pollutants in the air we breathe, of highly toxic pesticides and insecticides in agricultural practice and animal husbandry, there are a number of health hazards which are not sufficiently recognized or publicized by the health professions, but to which all food combiners should pay serious attention. *Otherwise they may not experience the full benefits of their new lifestyle*.

These health hazards include the dangers lurking in coffee, soft drinks and cola drinks; the unsuspected major illnesses arising from too much sugar (sucrose) in the diet; the perils in our drinking water; and the adverse effects on the chemical balance of the body by eating too much bread, be it white or whole-wheat.

On the other hand, attention should be paid to the great importance of eating as much fruit as can be afforded. Particular attention should be paid to the value of home-baked bread, and to the health-giving power of vitamin C (ascorbic acid); as a remarkable natural antibiotic and antioxidant it helps greatly to counteract many health hazards in our increasingly polluted environment.

Coffee

Most people regard coffee as a harmless drink, but it is known as a 'danger food'; the caffeine it contains can be a real troublemaker. Its harmful effects can include disturbance of the heart muscle, a too-high or too-low blood-pressure, PMT, insomnia, restlessness, constipation, increased risk of gastritis, lung and bladder cancer.

It can also have a serious effect on the mind, causing anxiety neurosis, irritability and depression.

Nutritionally, caffeine inhibits the body's absorption of minerals, promoting in particular a calcium loss through the kidneys. This loss is especially serious for women taking oral contraceptives; they are said to have an impaired elimination capacity for caffeine. Continued loss of calcium, moreover, can lead to hip fractures and the much dreaded osteoporosis in elderly people. All these harmful effects, alas, are never linked to coffee intake by coffee drinkers.

Heavy coffee drinkers should, therefore, be aware of these harmful effects and reduce their intake until they reach a moderate two to three cups per day. Milky coffee – is preferable to black coffee; the milk helps to buffer the caffeine and other toxins. Boston University Medical Centre warned in 1972 that people who drink more than five cups of coffee a day are twice as likely to suffer heart attacks as those who don't drink coffee at all.

Many people think that decaffeinated coffee is the answer to the coffee problem. But, as Barbara Griggs points out in *Zest for Life* (Ebury Press), decaffeinated coffee 'doesn't seem to be much less harmful than straight coffee, perhaps because caffeine is only one of many harmful nasties – powerful acids and dubious oils – in coffee. There are suspicions that the chemicals used to extract the caffeine may leave traces that are harmful to the body.'

For those wishing to reduce their daily coffee intake, try reducing the strength of the coffee infusion using Prewett's Instant Chicory, obtainable at Health Food shops. It is a soluble extract of roasted chicory root which has a surprisingly similar taste to real coffee – and is much cheaper! Reduce the usual amount of coffee powder by a dessertspoonful or so, according to the amount of coffee required, and compensate with a similar amount of chicory powder. Experiment with quantities, and also of water and/or milk, to obtain an acceptable brew. Using half nearly-boiling water to half hot milk gives a good result. The milk should not be overheated or allowed too near boiling point as this spoils the flavour of the coffee and reduces the nutritional value of the milk.

For those wishing to *give up* coffee drinking, instant chicory makes a very pleasant drink. It is good, too, as a cold drink, especially with a dribble of single cream. (*See Useful Addresses.*)

Infusing Coffee

The best way to make coffee, and by far the simplest, is by the Melita method, using special filter papers (unbleached by chlorine). These filter papers are said to hold back undesirable coffee oils and acids, roasting residues, and even the finest sediment. Coffee prepared this way is therefore less harmful than if prepared by other methods, and the flavour is excellent. But the coffee must be ground flour-fine, and should be Arabica not Robusta to get the best results. Finely ground coffee for use in filters is on sale in all supermarkets.

Cold-water Coffee

The following is a recipe which prevents (or greatly reduces) the extraction of caffeine from the coffee:

2 oz. (1 scant cup, American measure) finely ground coffee
2 pints (5 cups, American measure) cold water

Place the coffee in an earthenware, china or glass jug and add the water. Cover the jug and leave to steep for two days. During the first 24 hours stir up the grounds twice. At the end of two days the grounds will have sunk to the bottom of the jug and the coffee will be a clear liquid. Pour off the coffee carefully (or pass through a paper coffee filter) into another jug or bottle, and cover and cork it. To heat, place the amount required in an enamel pan, or other non-metal pan, but on no account let the coffee boil – this retains the flavour.

Made this way, the element which keeps some people awake at night is not extracted from the grounds. For best results, use bottled pure spring water. The amount of water used for the steeping must be adjusted to whatever strength of coffee is desired.

The drawback in making coffee this way is the difficulty in remembering to 'steep' a fresh lot of coffee grounds every two days!

Soft Drinks and Cola Drinks

Since the early eighties soft drink sales have doubled. This is cause for much concern as these drinks are virtually all sources of caffeine. In *The Daily Telegraph* of 5 October 1993, Christine Doyle questions the health repercussions of what she terms 'the flourishing caffeine culture', and she warns about the small but growing sale of high caffeine drinks.

'Caffeine,' writes Christine Doyle, 'is an acknowledged neuro stimulant and probably the world's most popular drug, present in coffee, tea, chocolate and cola drinks.' Surprisingly, it is even in a range of cold and headache remedies.

As caffeine promotes calcium loss in the body, and as children require an adequate amount of calcium to build strong teeth and bones, soft drinks and cola drinks should be taboo. They can be replaced with freshly prepared fruit drinks, or unsweetened, additive-free, bottled juices – organic preferably, but these, alas, are expensive.

Sugar (Sucrose)

Make no mistake about it – this is another 'deadly enemy' of health. Sugar steals both calcium and vitamin B from the body. Moreover, it changes friendly bacteria in the intestines into harmful ones (so preventing the manufacture there of other necessary vitamins), and impairs all body function. Sugar is now linked to a large percentage of present-day diseases connected with the heart, arteries, liver, skin, muscles, blood, kidneys, nerves, bones, ovaries and colon.

The formidable list of sugar-linked diseases makes a complete nonsense of the sugar lobby's claim that sugar does no harm to health and is 'a healthy, natural part of our diet.'

Just how unnatural sugar is can best be seen by the unnatural speed with which it is absorbed into the bloodstream, where it raises the blood sugar level too high for safety. In order to cope with this flow of sugar the pancreas pours out too much insulin, bringing the blood sugar level too low for safety, creating a metabolic paradox known as 'low blood sugar' or hypoglycaemia.

It is at this stage that the sugar addicts feel tired and weary, and firmly convinced that they *must* have some more sugar to give themselves energy. Thus a vicious cycle is begun and repeated over and over again. The resulting see-sawing between high and low blood sugar levels imposes a pathogenic strain on the pancreas and this, warns Surgeon Capt. T.L. Cleave in *The Saccharine Disease*, 'is the essential cause of (maturity-onset) diabetes'.

Digestion is designed to liberate nutrients *slowly* into the bloodstream in order to prevent overloading the system with a surfeit of energy foods at any one time. Naturally-occurring sugar, for example in an apple, is released slowly into the bloodstream, creates no see-sawing between high and low blood sugar levels, and does not contribute to diabetes.

It is highly significant that there has been a great increase in diabetes in the last 200 years, and a con-current increase in the consumption of sugar. Sugar is everywhere, even in savoury foods such as beef burgers, baked beans, sausages, tomato soup and tomato ketchup. The average consumption of sugar per head per annum is now about 100 lb. (50 kg)! Two hundred years ago, in Europe, it was only about 4 lb. (2 kg) per head per annum. Health seekers should beware of sugar and restrict it to very occasional use.

Honey – preferably from non-sugar-fed bees – is very helpful in solving culinary sweetening problems.

Honey is a remarkable food and has been known as such for thousands of years. But it is, like sugar, a 'concentrated carbohydrate' and therefore not compatible with acid fruits and proteins. But if you must have some sweetening in your salad dressings and fruit salads, for example, then by all means use honey – in strict moderation. Too much honey could be almost as harmful as too much sugar.

It is good to know that honey, like fruits, has an alkaline reaction in the body. In *The Complete Book of Food and Nutrition* (Rodale), J. I. Rodale writes about honey: 'Even though it is sweet, it contains, like fruit, certain organic acids which react in the body's chem-istry by producing alkalinity.'

It is not sufficiently known that honey is an excellent natural antiseptic, and for a short time in the 1970s it was used in the Berkshire Hospital, Reading, for dressing wounds and cuts, but was soon replaced by other dressings that were less 'messy'!

Water – the Perils in the Tap

Most of us take water for granted; it is something that is very much on tap, so to speak. That it can contribute to ill-health is seldom suspected by its trusting users.

Alas, there are many dangers lurking in our drinking water today, such as:

Lead: Regarded as the most serious one, and a well-known poison. According to Fred Pearce, former editor of *New Scientist*, pregnant women and babies whose bottle feeds are made up with tap water, are particularly at risk. In *Country Living* of September 1993, he warns that even low levels of lead can affect the development of young children.

Chlorine: Added to most water supplies to kill bacteria. But it can react with organic matter in the water to form what are called trihalomethanes (THMs) – suspected of being toxic and sometimes cancer-forming. In *The American Journal of Public Health* in July 1992, the by-products of chlorination were linked to cancer of the bladder, rectum and colon.

Chlorine is now regarded as one of the major health hazards of our age. Sensitive people should not indulge in long soaks in the bath; during a 'chlorine-high' period the immune system could be knocked down for days or weeks.

Aluminium sulphate: Added in small amounts to water by water companies as a floculant, to remove tiny floating particles that sometimes make water brown. Fred Pearce reports that a study in *The Lancet* in 1989 implicated aluminium in water as a possible cause of Alzheimer's disease. Because of concern on the part of water users, some water companies are now using iron sulphate instead.

Pesticides and nitrates: Used in agriculture, they seep from treated fields into underground water tables. 'Concentrations are low', writes Fred Pearce, 'but nobody knows whether, if drunk over many years, these chemicals could be dangerous.' High levels in the past have caused 'blue baby syndrome' – an oxygen deficiency in the baby's blood.

In the four years leading up to 1993, Friends of the Earth discovered that up to 16 million people in England and Wales had received tap water which contained illegally high levels of pesticides.

Despite the water companies' splendidly scientific processing of our drinking water – often against fearful odds – we may therefore be drinking a cocktail of small quantities of pesticides, the health effects of which, over many years, are unknown.

The inherent dangers of tap water, briefly outlined above, warrant providing a reliable water filter at the kitchen sink. Also a good bottled spring water, for drinking and cooking. It is important that this bottled water should have a *low* mineral content; water is not a good source of minerals as these are in 'inorganic' form and difficult for the body to utilize. Even more important, it should have a low fluoride content, not more than 0.2 parts per million (ppm), preferably 0.1 ppm.

A low fluoride content is imperative; fluoride is a poison and is classified as such by pharmacy laws, along with arsenic, lead and cyanide. Nevertheless, a fluoride compound is used to fluoridate water supplies, *mistakenly* to prevent dental decay in children's teeth.

Alas, once again, it is pregnant women and babies who are particularly at risk. *Fluoride should never be prescribed for pregnant women*; it 'locks up' magnesium, a deficiency of which can seriously inhibit respiratory enzymes which are essential for the oxygen-carrying capacity of the baby's blood. A deficiency of oxygen in the cells is regarded as one of the major causes of birth defects, Down's Syndrome, and infant mortality. It is, therefore, not surprising that inner Birmingham, long fluoridated, has been reported as having the highest infant death rate in England. Moreover, findings at the Brompton Hospital, West London, have indicated that a deficiency of oxygen in the baby's blood could be a cause of *cot death*. This was reported as a 'major breakthrough' by *Thames News, ITV*, in September 1985.

Especially at risk are bottle-fed babies whose feeds are reconstituted with fluoridated water. World experts are warning that they could be exposed to *eight times the recommended dose of fluoride*. It is, therefore, imperative that all bottle-fed babies in fluoridated areas should be supplied with a (low fluoride) bottled water by the DSS.

Especially at risk, also, are the elderly. The *Journal of the American Medical Association* (1990–1992) has reported a greater incidence of hip fractures in the UK, and also in the US. Fluoride treatment of

osteoporosis patients has also resulted in higher hip
fracture rates (the *New England Journal of Medicine*,
1990). Moreover, there is now clear evidence that
fluoridation causes *cancer* (*Fluoride the Ageing Factor*,
Dr John Viamougiannis, Health Action Press, 1993).

Fluoridation is without a doubt '*the greatest medical
fraud of the century*' according to Ivan Lawrence, QC,
MP (Hansard, 6 March 1980, Col. 772).

The Question of Fruit After Meals

Some recent versions of food combining recommend
that no fruit should be eaten after a protein or starch
meal. The argument is that the digestion of the fruit –
which is quick when eaten on its own – is retarded by
the slower digesting proteins and starches, resulting in
a fermentation.

This rule greatly lessens the enjoyment of the meal
for most people, and this enjoyment is essential for its
full digestion and benefit, according to Dr Hay. Such a
rule, moreover, where the main protein meal of the day
is concerned, can result in a somewhat 'thin' and
unsatisfying meal which, both psychologically and
gastronomically, does nothing to encourage a 'lifelong'
adherence to the diet. It should be remembered that
'a too strict regimen is a wearisome malady'.

Also, this rule appreciably reduces the amount of
fruit eaten during the day, especially the amount of
citrus fruits eaten. These, in correct combination, help
more than any other fruit to increase the vital alkaline
reserve of the body. According to Professor Derek
Bryce-Smith, citrus fruits also help to promote the

absorption of zinc – an all-important mineral – of which lean meat is a major source.

Fruit, ideally, should be eaten at every meal. Between meal fruit snacks, as recommended in some diets, are not always practical for many people. In conversation with Dr Hay many years ago, he insisted that he had invented no new or cranky diet; he had merely adapted one which was founded on ancient physiological laws which had once been known but long forgotten. These laws were observed around the time of Christ by a religious sect known as the Essenes, and came to light through translation from Aramaic and Slavonic manuscripts by Edmond Bordeaux Szekely in *The Essene Gospel of Peace* (the International Biogenic Society, 1981).

All Dr Hay did, he affirmed, was to present these ancient laws in a form that would be practical and enjoyable. He warned, moreover, that unless the diet was as practical as possible, eliminating unnecessary or punishing rules, a too-self-conscious preoccupation with food and with one's health, could result.

I have now been living by Dr Hay's precepts, promoting them and proving their truth beyond doubt, *for over 63 years*. It is of particular significance, therefore, that during this time I received countless letters from food combining enthusiasts whose health problems were resolved with remarkable speed, and whose excess weight rolled off just as speedily – without even trying to slim – *despite eating fruit after both starch and protein meals*.

These facts speak for themselves and should resolve any doubts about eating fruit to complete these meals. As Dr Linus Pauling – two-time Nobel

Laureate – believed: 'A successful treatment is one that will be adhered to, year after year. To achieve such continual compliance *the diet should appeal to the appetite.*' [added emphasis]

Vitamin C (Ascorbic acid)

In compiling this section I wish to acknowledge the help and inspiration from *How to Live Longer and Feel Better* by Dr Linus Pauling, world-renowned for his achievements in the laboratory and in the cause of world peace; *You Don't Have to be Sick* by the famous Australian doctor, Phyllis Cilento; *Every Second Child* by another famous Australian doctor, Archie Kalokerinos who, working among aboriginal children in Western New South Wales, reduced the high death rate among aboriginal babies and children from almost 'every second child' to practically zero by the use of vitamin C; *The Healing Factor: Vitamin C Against Disease*, the epoch-making book by Dr Irwin Stone, and *Vitamin C – The Master Nutrient* – by Dr Sandra Goodman, a leading authority on this vitamin.

The discovery of vitamins nearly 80 years ago, and the recognition of their momentous significance in a healthy diet, was one of *the most important contributions to health that was ever made.*

'Of equal importance,' wrote Dr Linus Pauling, 'was the recognition about 20 years ago that the optimum intakes of several of the vitamins, far larger than the usually recommended intakes, lead to further improvements in health, greater protection against many diseases, and enhanced effectiveness in the therapy of diseases. The potency of vitamin C and other vitamins is explained by the new understanding that they function principally by strengthening the natural protective mechanisms of the body, especially the immune system.'

Unfortunately, despite all the published evidence of vitamin C's great value, the larger doses recommended by Linus Pauling antagonized the US federal medical agencies, and medicos in high places, who all continued to deny that vitamin C had any value. As a result, many 'incorrect' statements found their way into pamphlets, authoritative reference books and textbooks – proof indeed that their authors had failed to understand or assess correctly the published evidence about vitamin C.

The reader is, no doubt, familiar with some of these incorrect statements: 'Excess vitamin C causes gouty arthritis'; 'Large doses of vitamin C cause infertility and a tendancy to miscarriage'; 'High doses of vitamin C destroy substantial amounts of vitamin B12 in food'; and 'Users of high doses of vitamin C develop kidney stones'. These 'myths' are thoroughly addressed in Dr Sandra Goodman's book in the chapter aptly called 'Myths and Facts' (pp 17–31).

But as Dr Archie Kalokerinos has pointed out: 'The so-called "dangerous" side-effects of vitamin C – so often quoted – do not, in reality, exist.'

We Can't Make Our Own Vitamin C

Although nearly all mammals manufacture ascorbic acid in the liver from the blood sugar (glucose), man cannot do so. Millions of years ago, a mutation (probably) occurred in our ancestral species of primates which prevented their ability to manufacture the one enzyme which will turn glucose into ascorbic acid, or vitamin C. In this way Dr Irwin Stone explains what probably happened to our evolving primaeval ancestors and the reason for our inability, today, to make our own vitamin C.

We are, therefore, dependent on outside sources for our vitamin C – mainly fruit, vegetables and salad foods. But for optimum health and protection against many diseases, far larger quantities are required than even foods with a high vitamin C content can provide. Fortunately, through the original work of Dr Szent Gyorgyi, who isolated vitamin C in 1928, and that of Walter Howarth, who synthesized it soon afterwards (and for which both men received Nobel Prizes in 1937), we are able to buy as much as we need of vitamin C, 'essentially the same ascorbic acid that we cannot manufacture ourselves,' as Phyllis Cilento points out.

Vitamin C Fulfils Many Vital Functions in the Human Body

The most definitely established of all its functions, is that of assisting in the formation of collagen – the cement that holds the bricks of the body together. Collagen is of supreme importance; it is the most abundant of the body's proteins and makes up 30 per cent of them. 'When vitamin C is deficient,' writes Phyllis Cilento, 'the body literally comes apart at the seams.' *A deficiency contributes to the ageing process.*

Vitamin C helps, and protects against, many conditions and diseases:

Diabetes: Researchers over the years have shown that ascorbic acid actually improves the action of insulin and makes it possible to get the same effect with smaller doses. 'Diabetics should take vitamin C – say 1,000 mg to 4,000 mg a day, not only to activate insulin, but to prevent infections to which they are particularly prone,' recommends Phyllis Cilento.

Asthma: In the 1930s and 1940s a great deal of research on the role of vitamin C in asthma produced conflicting results for two reasons. *First*, doses were too small and too infrequent to affect the allergic condition; *Second*, insufficient doses seemed to make the symptoms worse. Then, when effective drugs were introduced – antihistamines, cortisone, antibiotics – all interest in vitamin C and asthma flagged.

This interest is only just being revived. Phyllis Cilento writes: 'It is now recognized that the protective effect of vitamin C, as with other allergies, is dose-dependent, and large or megadoses are needed to scotch asthma attacks and to keep the asthmatic free from a habitual allergic response to the particular allergens to which he is susceptible.' She uses large doses of vitamin C – 6 to 10 g per day (more conveniently taken as sodium ascorbate powder) to maintain chronic asthmatics free from attacks at all times. She warns, of course, that their particular allergic substances should be avoided as far as possible, and that their diet should be well balanced, with plenty of fresh, non-additive foods. It would appear that the excellent results asthma sufferers experience on Hay principles could be increased still further for optimum health with vitamin C supplementation.

Arthritis and rheumatism: In the early tests of

vitamin C to alleviate arthritis or rheumatism, far too
small doses off vitamin C were used, as in the early
treatment of asthma. Reports since the 1940s, however,
have shown excellent results with large doses of 4 g
(1 g four times daily), to 8 g to 12 g a day. Again, a
well-balanced diet is essential, say both Linus Pauling
and Phyllis Cilento. If the condition is especially stubborn, supplementation with vitamins A, E and the B
complex is recommended. On a food combining diet,
remarkably, arthritis symptoms are recorded as alleviated or resolved – *without supplementation*. Results,
however, would be speeded up, and health generally
improved, with added vitamin C.

Bacterial and viral infections: Vitamin C in strong
concentrations destroys bacteria and viruses, or
prevents their growth, and *acts as a natural antibiotic*.

In *You Don't Have to be Sick*, the effects of high-
dose vitamin C on a number of other diseases and
conditions are recorded. These include hay fever and
other allergies, heart and artery diseases, herpes, cot
deaths, ulcers, cataracts and mental troubles. Even the
effect of vitamin C on the ailments of dogs and cats
is included: 'The treatment of colds, distemper and
kidney disease is improved by doses of vitamin C
several times a day, about 100 to 200 mg at a time.'
Moreover, many dog and cat owners have found that
their pets improve in health and vitality and their coats
grow glossy when some vitamin C is added to their
diet.

Also, in *Vitamin C – The Master Nutrient* – which
brings together hundreds of published studies –
Sandra Goodman discusses the use of vitamin C in the
prevention and treatment of a host of health problems,

including arthritis, cancer, heart disease, diabetes and AIDS.

Those in special need of extra vitamin C include:

- Alcoholics and heavy drinkers;
- Cigarette smokers;
- Women on the pill;
- Workers in garages and service stations;
- Farmers and horticulturalists;
- People subject to colds, coughs and bronchitis;
- Expectant and nursing mothers;
- Those living or working near main roads.

In need of vitamin C, also, are physical fitness fans. In his foreword to Phyllis Cilento's book, Dr Archie Kalokerinos warns: 'To those who believe in the advantages of physical fitness, vitamin C is of extreme importance. To exercise strenuously without sufficient vitamin C can result in ill-health or death. For some "sufficient" could be a great deal, so care should be taken to provide this.'

The very next day after the above paragraph was written, *The Daily Mail* reported the death of a model from a brain haemorrhage, after she had collapsed on an exercise bike. Had she known about vitamin C she might still be alive today.

Of the future of vitamin C, Phyllis Cilento believes: 'that the awareness of the value and life-saving properties of vitamin C (in one of its forms) will be the most important breakthrough of this century and will ensure better health for thousands, and freedom from many of the diseases that now beset us.'

Antioxidants, Free Radicals and Vitamin C

It would appear that this 'important breakthrough' has begun. Vitamin C is now also being hailed as a potent *antioxidant*, along with beta-carotene (the precursor of vitamin A) and vitamin E. New evidence has revealed that antioxidants can reduce the risk of a number of diseases, such as coronary heart disease, rheumatoid arthritis, Parkinson's disease, cataracts, AIDS and some types of cancer.

In her excellent article in 'Health Care' (*Sunday Times*, 31 October 1993), Sarah Stacey describes how antioxidants work – by mopping up 'free radicals' which are now regarded as the underlying cause of many degenerative diseases and of the ageing process itself. A 'free radical', explains Sarah, 'is any molecule in the body which carries an unpaired electron . . . our cells produce thousands of free radicals every day and some are necessary for life. In excess, however, these randy single molecules cause havoc as they rush around looking for a mate to pair with, in order to produce the oxidizing process which can lead to cellular damage and disease.'

It is a sobering fact that the great increase in ill-health during the latter part of this century is now being blamed by experts on the proliferation of free radicals caused by countless pollutants in our environment. Helpfully, 'the best known antioxidants', points out Sarah Stacey, 'are beta-carotene and vitamins C and E. Back-up troops include the so-called 'scavenger' minerals – selenium, copper, zinc and manganese.'

Supplementation with these vitamins and minerals

would seem to be common sense. Many doctors and dieticians, however, still maintain that such supplementation is unnecessary, as a balanced diet provides adequate supplies of nutrients. But no matter how good the diet, or how much fresh fruit and vegetables are consumed daily, it would be impossible to eat enough to provide the megadoses necessary for therapeutic use. Anthony Diplock, Professor of Biochemistry at Guy's and St Thomas's Hospitals Medical School, believes that the only way to achieve preventive levels of antioxidants is by taking supplements. He also believes, 'that in the interests of helping protect the country's population from the two biggest killers of our time (heart disease and cancer) . . . the Government should provide free antioxidant supplementation, in the same way as it does vitamin drops for babies.' This would possibly be far less costly for the Health Ministry than their present bill for drugs and hospital care.

Professor Diplock recommends daily: 10 to 15mg of beta-carotene, 150 to 200mg of Vitamin C, 50 to 100mg of vitamin E, and 50 to 60 microgrammes of selenium – all these amounts, it should be noted, are way above the Government's recommended daily allowance.

Linus Pauling, on the other hand, recommends much higher daily doses of vitamins: Vitamin C: 6g; Vitamin E: 400 international units (iu), 800 iu, or indeed as much as 16 thousand iu (as deemed necessary according to personal circumstance); Vitamin B: One or two Super B tablets; Vitamin A: one 25-thousand IU tablet; and one multi-mineral tablet. He emphasizes that these amounts 'are firmly based on the new science of nutrition that has been developed only during recent years,' and that the difference between this new science and the old one, 'is the recognition that vitamins taken in the optimum amounts have far greater value than when taken in the usually recommended small amounts.' He also emphasizes that with the optimum intake of supplementary vitamins, 'there is no longer so much need to stress other dietary measures, such as decreasing the intake of animal fat and not eating eggs . . . and that the quality of life is enhanced when one is liberated from these dietary restrictions.'*

At long last the 'new science of nutrition' is being slowly but surely recognized as a necessary adjunct to medical care – in particular, the role of nutritional supplements. Regarding the use of these, Dr Walter Barker, Senior Research Fellow at the University of Bristol, writes emphatically:

> 'With the insight we now possess, it is a little short of negligence to offer medical care without nutritional care; in those cases where the significance of specific nutritional supplements in the treatment of illness has been shown in numerous research studies, failure to use such supplements alongside the medical treatment is arguably a serious negligence.

*As vitamins and minerals act together like the members of an orchestra, all should be included in the diet as far as possible – vitamin E in particular, when increasing vitamin C. It should be noted that dosage of vitamin C should be before, during or after meals – and *the daily dose should never be omitted*, even for one day, warns Dr Linus Pauling.

'For three of the great human killers, it has yet to be recognized that it is nutrition and the wider environment, in interaction, which have the primary responsibility for both the illness and any hope of their remediation.'

(Guest editorial: Health: State-of-the-Art, Vol. 1, Issue 1, See Recommended Reading)

The Cost of Supplementation

Supplementing the diet with vitamins and minerals, alas, is expensive, especially with these higher doses. *The Hay System, however, can appreciably reduce the cost.* This is undeniably suggested by the fact that the remarkable healings and ameliorations of a wide variety of conditions recorded in Chapter 3 were achieved without supplementation in most, if not all, cases.

There are two possible reasons for this: *First*, more nourishment is derived from properly combined foods. *Second*, the 'normal' alkalinity of the body fluids created by these foods is 'the most favourable for the action of vitamins', as Dr Dudley d'Avergne Wright pointed out in *Foods for Health and Healing* (Health Science Press).

Despite the benefits of food combining, however, every endeavour should be made to supplement the diet with vitamins and minerals, not only to achieve the optimum health, but also to help counteract the increasing pollution of the environment and the 'free radicals' which this creates. With regard to these, vitamin C is of particular importance, acting as it does as a powerful antioxidant. The cheapest way to buy it is in powder form as ascorbic acid or as 'calcium ascorbate', which tastes less acid (*See Useful Addresses*).

'Vitamin C and Cancer: The Irrefutable Evidence'

This is the title of an article by Sandra Goodman, PhD, in the *International Journal of Alternative and Complementary Medicine*, January 1994.

Sandra, the author of *Vitamin C – The Master Nutrient*, is a molecular biologist and earned her PhD at McGill University. Regarding the irrefutable evidence she writes:

'Hundreds of research studies published during the past decade alone attest to the monumental research effort mobilized to document the role of vitamin C in cancer prevention and treatment. Numerous books, each replete with hundreds of references, have been published over the years, documenting the vital role played by vitamin C in every body system function. For vitamin C is a potent antioxidant, immune modulator, integral to countless metabolic endocrine and neurological functions, vital for skin, bone, muscle and connective tissue.'

Sandra lists seven mechanisms whereby vitamin C's anti-cancer properties are brought about. It is sufficient to quote just three of these to understand how vitamin C affords such remarkable protection from cancer: It scavenges cancer-causing free radicals such as hydrogen peroxide to prevent lipid (fat) peroxidation and destruction of cells; it neutralizes carcinogenic chemicals such as nitrosamines and nitrites; it enhances lymphocyte function and rapid mobilization of phagocytes.

With all the evidence which massive new research has produced, vitamin C must now have achieved medical respectability, and Dr Linus Pauling must surely have won his long and arduous battle with professional hostility over his championing of this quite remarkable and versatile nutrient.

Since the foregoing paragraph was written, a television documentary in July 1994, confirmed that Dr Pauling was at long last seeing his work on vitamin C taken seriously, following discoveries that vitamin C not only acts as a potent antioxidant, but that large doses can extend the lifespan and lessen susceptibility to disease.

A month later, on 21 August, Dr Linus Pauling died at the age of 93. Obituaries in the daily press hailed him as one of the greatest scientists of the twentieth century, and one of the most important scientists of all time, along with Isaac Newton, Marie Curie and Albert Einstein. Dr Pauling was the only man to win two unshared Nobel prizes in different fields: In 1934 he was awarded the Nobel Prize for Chemistry, and in 1963, the Nobel Prize for Peace. He was a giant among men.

Bread – Once a Day Only

There are many different wholewheat breads on super-
market shelves today – such breads, thankfully, no
longer have a connotation of 'crankiness': but none can
compare with the home-baked variety, especially the
easy-to-make, no-knead bread, known for over 50 years
as 'The Grant Loaf'.

Until you have tasted such bread you don't know
how good wholewheat bread can be or what remarkable
things it can do for health, stamina and happiness.

Eating too much bread (or other 'concentrated
carbohydrate'), however, can have an adverse and
unsuspected effect on digestion and health, as a correspondent discovered some years ago:

'Though I have been a food reformer and vegetarian for the past 10 years or so, my health has
never been very good and I was very unhappy
about it because I wanted so much to tell people
around me of the benefits of food reform. You
have showed me my mistake – *an excess of starch*.
For me it was bread, wholewheat bread. As it was
'good for me' I simply indulged in it, *at every
meal and between meals*! I felt more and more tired
with no real 'joie de vivre'. The starch/protein
theory is, I am convinced, absolutely exact and
digestion seems much easier after only a week of
separating incompatible foods.'

A basic 'food combining' rule is that bread should
not be eaten more than once a day (except for those

doing strenuous manual labour!). There are two good reasons for this:

First: The minerals in bread, being mostly phosphatic, are acid-forming in tendency – that is, when burned up by the digestive system, they leave behind an acid residue. Too much acid residue lowers the resistance to disease and unbalances the body chemistry.

Bread is, therefore, listed as an 'acid-forming' food. The dangers of the predominance of the acid-forming foods were clearly stressed by Professor E.V. McCollum, internationally known authority on nutrition at Johns Hopkins University:

> 'If the acids predominate strongly over the basis regularly for considerable periods of time, the alkalinity of the blood will be reduced and acidosis will result. Some eminent physicians now believe that the diseases of the blood which are responsible for high blood-pressure, kidney disease, gangrene and apoplexy (all of which are common side-effects of diabetes) are the result of prolonged injury due to eating excessive amounts of acid-forming foods.'

Second: Eating bread at a main meal – especially at a protein meal, reduces the appetite, and the space, for a sufficiency of the accompanying vegetables and salad foods and fruit which are necessary for a well-balanced diet, and which, moreover, are an even better source than bread of the 'soluble' and 'insoluble' fibres which help to lower blood cholesterol and prevent some of the diseases of Western civilization.

The Grant Loaf

It was an accidental discovery – even an instinctive one, perhaps – which was responsible for prompting the recipe for this no-kneading bread.

After I had been making bread for about six months, I discovered to my amazement that I had been missing out what is usually considered the most important part of the whole process – I had not been kneading the bread after the first rising!

In spite of this, my bread was delicious, moist and chewy, with the full flavour of the whole wheat grain. I could only conclude that it was, perhaps, because of this very omission that my bread was considered by both family and visitors to be so specially good.

When making two loaves for the next baking, I kneaded one loaf and left the other unkneaded. The loaves were then baked in the same oven for the same length of time, and were cut for testing at the same time. The kneaded loaf tasted very ordinary and not at all 'moreish'. The unkneaded loaf smelt inviting and its taste was delicious and *very* 'moreish'. The difference between the two loaves was astonishing.

My own explanation for this, for what it is worth, is that the air spaces, formed in the dough by the working yeast, may contain some essential oils, vitamins, or other qualities of the wheat; that the yeast itself may confer an essential something to the bread. When the air spaces are broken open during the kneading, these qualities escape and are lost. I have had this story confirmed by an old, retired baker. On no account, he affirmed, should wholewheat bread be kneaded, but white bread, on the other hand, can be kneaded without loss, having possibly lost much of its goodness and qualities in the milling process.

This no-kneading bread has been popular with home bakers for over 50 years since it was published in *Your Daily Bread* (Faber & Faber). It has been quoted in many articles, and included in a number of cookery books on bread, such as *The Sunday Times Book of Real Bread* by Michael Bateman and Heather Maisner; *English Bread and Yeast Cookery* by Elizabeth David; *The Good Cook BREADS* by the editors of Time Life Books; *Thoughts on Feeding* by Lionel James Picton, OBE; *Nature's Plan for Your Health* by Thomas Bartram; and *Delia Smith's The Complete Cookery Course*. Delia Smith writes (of her own version of my recipe): 'Although it is quick and easy, it has a wonderful, wholesome home-made flavour. For those of us who simply don't have the time for kneading, knocking down and proving, this loaf is an absolute gem and the one that I, personally, make most often.' Delia also demonstrated the Grant Loaf on one of her television programmes.

Your Daily Bread brought me a stream of letters for many years. They came from enthusiastic Grant Loafers, as they called themselves, from all over the world. Two letters in particular made an indelible impression on my memory.

The first was from an Australian businessman whose work took him to small camps throughout some of the most inhospitable parts of the Australian continent. The men in these camps were boring artesian wells in various places in the cattle country. When he discovered them baking their own bread, he introduced them, with great success, to the Grant no-kneading method; it was so much quicker and easier to make than their own method and tasted so much nicer. He ended his letter: 'So the wise words you have written are bearing fruit in a most distant land . . . should you ever find yourself in Australia, I can say you will find *Welcome* on the mat!'

The second letter was not addressed to me, but was the response to a *Housewife* magazine competition (August, 1949) to describe 'The Best Thing I Ever Made'.

The winner of the first prize wrote: 'What, in my 36 years of life, has given me the most satisfaction to make? The Grant Loaf. I was on the point of giving up *Housewife* when the recipe for the Grant Loaf appeared in it.' She then admitted she was sick of wonderful housewives who managed homes and children so miraculously; she had no children and no proper home. She and her husband lived in a one-room unconverted sports pavilion – no lighting, no fireplace, and, although heated by two radiators, draughty and comfortless, with no room for a cooking stove. They both read about the 'Grant bread' and decided to try it when they had a decent home. She wrote:

'Why wait? An oven on an iron stand above the Primus cooked two lovely loaves. No more shop bread for us. My outlook changed. If I could bake bread I could do other things. I baked cakes, I bottled fruit. That one-roomed dwelling became a home, and even achieved some comfort. At least we didn't have to share bathrooms and kitchens. We have moved now. I have a home and a child. I learned to make the best of things to hand instead of fretting for the unattainable.'

What better proof than this letter of the ease with which the Grant Loaf can be made – even in daunting conditions – and the quite 'unexpected benefits' it can produce?

THE GRANT LOAF

(Note: All the following bread recipes freeze well.)

Metric (Imperial)	*American*
1.35kg (3 lb.) stone ground wholewheat flour	12 cupsful stone ground wholewheat flour
2 teaspoonsful or less sea salt	2 teaspoonsful or less sea salt
1.2 litres (2 pints) water at blood heat (98.4°F/37°C)	5 cupsful water at blood heat (98.4°F/37°C)
3 level teaspoonsful dried yeast	3 level teaspoonsful dried yeast
2 level teaspoonsful Barbados sugar, honey or black molasses	2 level teaspoonsful Barbados sugar, honey or black molasses

1. Mix the salt with the flour (in very cold weather warm flour slightly to take off the chill).
2. Place 3 tablespoonsful of the water in a cup,

sprinkle the dried yeast on top and leave for 2 minutes.

3. Add the sugar, honey or molasses. Leave for a further 10–15 minutes by which time there should be a thick creamy froth.

4. Make a well in the centre of the flour and pour in the yeast mixture and the rest of the water.

5. Mix well – by hand is best – for a minute or so, working from sides to middle until the dough feels elastic and leaves the sides off the mixing bowl clean. Flours tend to vary in how much water they take up – the dough should be slippery.

6. Divide the dough into three 1 litre (2 pint/5 cup) bread tins which have been warmed and greased.

7. Put the tins in a warm (not hot) place, cover with a clean cloth and leave for about 20 minutes or until the dough is within 1 cm (½ in.) of the top of the tins.

8. Bake in a fairly hot oven, 400°F/200°C (Gas Mark 6), for 35 to 40 minutes. If the loaf sounds hollow when the top is knocked, it is done.

Quantities for One Loaf:

Metric (Imperial)	*American*
450g (1 lb.) stoneground wholewheat flour	4 cupsful stoneground wholewheat flour
½ teaspoonful sea salt	½ teaspoonful sea salt
360ml (13–14 fl. oz.) water at blood heat (98.4°F/37°C)	1¾ cupsful water at blood heat (98.4°F/37°C)

1½ level teaspoonsful
dried yeast
1 teaspoonful Barbados
sugar, honey or black
molasses

1½ level teaspoonsful
dried yeast
1 teaspoonful Barbados
sugar, honey or black
molasses

Variations on the Grant Loaf:

The Bran-plus Loaf

1. Substitute 40g (1½ oz./⅓ cupful) fresh unprocessed
   bran for 40g (1½ oz./⅓ cupful) wholewheat flour in
   every 450g (1 lb./4 cupsful)
2. Method – as for the Grant Loaf.

The Gordon Grant Loaf

1. Substitute 25g (1oz./¼ cupful) medium cut oatmeal
   for 25g (1 oz./¼ cupful) wholewheat flour in every
   450g (1 lb./4 cupsful)
2. Before baking the loaves, sprinkle sesame seeds
   thickly on top of the dough and press them down
   gently to make them adhere.
3. Method – as for the Grant Loaf.

Note: The oatmeal enhances the lovely nutty flavour
of the bread and increases its moisture-keeping quality.
(This is what my husband has done to my loaf! – D.G.)

Wholeness

—— ❧ ——

Man shall not live by bread alone, . . .

(Matt. 4:4)

Some years ago, in an outstanding TV science review, a spot of blood was shown under an electron microscope. It provided an amazing live 'close-up' of red blood cells, with some white cells and invading streptococci. One was forcibly struck with the impression that the white cells seemed to know exactly what they were doing, where they were going, and that they were prompted by some guiding force.

At first only the red blood cells and streptococci could be seen. The latter were attacking the red blood cells which 'popped' and disappeared on contact with the invaders. Then on to the field rushed the rescue squad, the white blood cells, pushing and shoving determinedly past the immobile red ones, pursuing the streptococci and engulfing them in one mouthful. Soon all the invaders were disposed of.

This extraordinary display left one with the overwhelming conviction of having witnessed the life-force in action.

We must nourish this life-force. Dr Hay never forgot to stress the importance of nourishing the whole being – physical, mental and spiritual. He particularly stressed the importance of spiritual health, and this involves not only right eating but also right thinking.

The Power of Thought and the Whole Being

Ralph Waldo Trine, in his famous and inspiring book, *In Tune With the Infinite*[1] has much to say about the power of thought: that thought is not an abstract thing but 'a vital living force, the most vital, subtle, and invisible force there is in the universe.'

He warns that the effects of the mind upon the body are far greater than generally realized. The mind and body are closely linked, and '. . . what happens in the mind is inevitably reflected in the health or disease of the body. Thus, a poor diet and negative outlook can weaken the immune system, which increases one's susceptibility to illness'; negative thoughts such as fear and worry, for instance '. . . have the effects of closing up the channels of the body, so that the lifeforces flow in a slow and sluggish manner.' He goes on to affirm that hope and tranquillity open up these channels.

Nourishing the Life-force

Ralph Waldo Trine's remarkable book was published at the end of the last century in 1887. Nearly 100 years later, in 1986, another remarkable book was published, *Nourishing the Life Force*[2] containing the same inspiring truths. Its authors, Richard and Mary Jafolla, say in their introduction that they set out to write a treatise on healing and health, with special emphasis on 'nourishing the life-force', and working with it to help overcome specific health challenges. As did Ralph Trine, they too stress the importance to health of right thinking, but with an added special emphasis on right eating and the value of vitamin and mineral supplements. Also, like Ralph Trine, they stress that the life-force is universal – omnipresent – and they describe it in this beautiful passage:

> 'This mysterious life force in our bodies is the same universal force that holds the planets in their orbits, causes the tides to rise and fall, brings forth the sequoia from the tiny seed, and propels an amoeba through a drop of water. And the direction of this force, this spirit, is always towards good, an eternal quest for perfection and the awareness of the complete unity of all life.'

This omnipresent force is clearly evident on every hand in what is commonly referred to as the healing power of nature, in the seemingly magical way, for instance, that cuts and bruises can heal by themselves. It would appear to be evident, also, in the remarkable healings recorded in Chapters 3 and 4. Nowhere, however, does it appear so *visibly evident* than in the tiny, delicately perfect frond of a fern which has pushed its way up to the light through a solid asphalt pavement.

The Newer Knowledge of Nutrition

In 1937, Sir Robert McCarrison, whose original research into deficiency diseases has been an inspiration to researchers and laymen alike throughout the world, affirmed in his *Cantor Lectures*[3]:

> 'The newer knowledge of nutrition is, I am convinced, the greatest advance in medicine since the days of Lister ... when physicians, medical officers of health, and the lay public learn to apply the principles which this newer knowledge of nutrition has to impart ... then will this knowledge do for medicine which asepsis has done for surgery.'

Again, in December 1957, Dr Hugh Sinclair, Fellow of Magdalen College, Oxford, affirmed in his World Health Day speech:

> 'The new science of nutrition will shed much needed light on one of the most fundamental, widespread, urgent and inadequately managed problems in the whole domain of human welfare. For nutrition has now become the most important single environmental factor affecting health in every country in the world.'[4]

Despite these powerful pronouncements regarding the importance of nutrition to human welfare, nutrition in the context of sensible dietary choice (rather than that of biochemistry or medicine) is not yet adequately taught in medical and dental schools. In fact, a review some years ago of medical education by the General Medical Council *did not recognize nutrition as a mandatory subject*.

As Dr Kenneth Vickery has observed: 'It is astonishing that scientific man has reached such an advanced state of twentieth century knowledge without having grasped the ecological message of soil, food and health.' Unfortunately, this message gets sparse emphasis from the medical profession as a whole in its daily practice, and nutrition is not being taught effectively to medical students, midwives, health visitors, advisers on parenthood or, especially, to school children and school teachers.

Meantime, Britain becomes no healthier, despite more hospitals, more drugs, and an ever more costly Health Service. Britain, in fact, has been called 'the sick man, woman and child of Europe'.[5] Heart attack, Britain's largest killer, is reported to claim an average 270 people each day. Especially disturbing is the new phenomenon of the incidence in young children of diseases, such as cancer, that formerly mainly attacked adults or the very elderly. Cancer is reported to be the second most common cause of death in children today. During the past three decades childhood eczema has doubled[6] and childhood insulin-dependent diabetes has increased sixfold[7]. Adolescent obesity is also a problem (as it is for adults), and according to Dr Walter Barker, Director of the Child Health Development Programme at Bristol University, there is 'a tremendous amount of recurring illness, like diarrhoea and chest infections which shouldn't be there.'

The Government's own report *Fit for Life*[8] in 1976, revealed that there is an alarmingly high infant death rate in Britain compared to other countries, and much acute illness in childhood. Recently, moreover, there have been reports of 'clusters' of incidence of thalidomide-type deformities in newborn babies, for which, at the time of writing, no positive explanation has been found.

Moreover, according to *Health of the Nation*, in 1991, there were nearly twice as many deaths from cancer as in 1931, and nearly twice as many deaths from circulatory diseases![9] Recent figures, however, from the World Health Organisation of the alarming increase since 1920 of civilization diseases in Europe (published in *Raum und Zeit* September/October 1994) suggest that the *Health of the Nation* death rates for cancer and circulatory diseases are somewhat on the conservative side.

Nutrient-deficient Food and Asocial Behaviour

Meantime, also, the crimewave plaguing Britain becomes increasingly violent, despite all the benefits of the Welfare State. Teachers are viciously attacked in class; women, even the very elderly, are brutally assaulted; small children are murdered or raped by other children hardly out of kindergarten; robberies with violence and vandalism are now commonplace; nearly every day a murder somewhere is reported, and juvenile delinquency is increasingly vicious and alarming.

Among the many classic explanations for crime and juvenile delinquency, in the past were genetics, lack of parental discipline, lack of education, poor housing and broken homes. But never has there been any mention that the present-day diet of refined carbohydrates – white flour, white sugar and all foods made with them – and chemicalized, processed foods, could be a large contributing factor to juvenile delinquency and adult crime of all kinds.

One far-sighted doctor, however, who drew attention to this serious oversight, was Aubrey Westlake. In his illuminating book, *Life Threatened*[10], he wrote:

'Never anywhere in the interminable discussions, conferences, symposiums, committees of investigation, etc., etc., have I seen it suggested that present-day diet might be one of the major factors in juvenile delinquency and adolescent waywardness.'

And he pointed to these evils running parallel to the increasing adulteration and refinement of our food.

Since the early part of this century there have been a number of researchers investigating the relationship between such food and asocial behaviour. Outstanding among these is the eminent American dentist, Dr Weston Price. During his world-wide investigation of about 14 primitive peoples living on their traditional diets of unrefined, unprocessed foods, he made the interesting observation that they all had two striking characteristics in common – *a high standard of behaviour* and the virtual absence of violence or crime in any form. When these primitive peoples came into contact with civilization, however, *one generation* on 'civilized' processed refined food was sufficient to cause happy, kindly people to turn into morose, discontented, quarrelsome ones. It was also sufficient to cause physical degeneration – poor skeletal structure, narrow dental arches, and dental caries. Dr Price's book, *Nutrition and Physical Degeneration*[11], is a classic of its kind.

Chemical Children[12], by Dr Peter Mansfield and Dr Jean Munro – two outstanding investigators – is another classic of its kind. It reveals from their combined clinical experience that our processed, refined foods and our chemically polluted air, water and soil are causing massive and serious health problems in children as well as hyperactive and psychiatric disorders which can disrupt both schooling and family life[*]. *Chemical Children* should be made compulsory reading for all parents, social workers and government health bodies.

Another outstanding investigator is Dr Richard Mackarness[13], a well-known pioneer in Britain of 'clinical ecology' until he emigrated to Australia some years ago. His now widely-told story of Michael well demonstrates the often disastrous effects on children of today's 'jitterbug diet'. It was told by Dr Mackarness at the International Congress of Social Psychiatry in London in 1964.

Michael was a small boy of seven who was so viciously naughty that his mother and teachers could

---

[*]Parents who need help with children who are hyperactive, have psychiatric or eating disorders, should contact The Hyperactive Society Children's Support Group (*see Useful Addresses, page 164*).

do nothing with him. His diet consisted mainly of sugar-high foods and refined carbohydrates – iced lollies, milk chocolate, cakes, biscuits, cornflakes and white bread. This mounted up to a serious deficiency of B vitamins, among other factors. Dr Mack (as he is affectionately called by his patients) replaced these deficiency foods with a sound diet of B-containing vitamins, such as 100 per cent wholewheat bread. Within the space of three days, Michael began to show great improvement. By the end of a week he was a normal and charming little boy!

To make sure, however, that Michael's mother was completely convinced of the effects of this new diet, Dr Mack put Michael back on his old one. In two days he was worse than ever and almost beyond control. His mother was then completely convinced and promptly returned him to his new diet with the same excellent results as before.

The sociologists and educators will have to pay attention to the question of food and its impact on the body and mind before the present situation becomes beyond control. There is much confirmatory evidence on this issue, and many medical authorities who would be happy to be consulted.

The educators must start the ball rolling. The first priority must be to start teaching children, from kindergarten to University, about properly constituted food and its potential for health, happiness and character. Most important of all, children must be taught *the difference between right and wrong*.

By an extraordinary coincidence, the very morning after the foregoing section was written, huge headlines in *The Daily Mail*, of 16 May 1994, revealed that the educators have indeed started the ball rolling: '*Classes in Morality: Children of five to learn clear values*'. The article, by Roy Massey, Education Correspondent, is so apt that it must be quoted at some length:

> 'Children as young as five are to attend classes in morality and manners. They will learn through stories, games and role play the difference between right and wrong in an effort to improve their behaviour and cut crime and vandalism.
>
> 'Pupils will be told to respect other people's property and feelings, to accept racial differences and be given examples of acceptable behaviour.
>
> 'The programme will be launched by Michael Howard who is expected to visit a South London primary school to see it in action . . .
>
> 'Ministers are concerned that too many youngsters are growing up without the necessary knowledge and experience to operate in a civilized society . . .
>
> 'Mark Seaton, Chairman of the Campaign for Real Education, said: 'Youngsters should be taught clear values such as the ten commandments. It is very important that they know the difference between right and wrong.'

The health educators deserve the highest commendation for putting into action the classes in morality devised by the newly formed Citizenship Foundation. Once again, however, any teaching about the fundamental need for a healthy diet seems to have been overlooked.

Survival

In order to survive, our chief task must be to free the world from its stranglehold of materialism. It is mainly because we have thrown overboard our spiritual values that the whole world is in its present state of turmoil.

There is cause for optimism, however. Science, so long at war with religion, may now be actually *affirming* religion. Since our newer knowledge of the atom, physicists have discovered that matter is not as solid as we had been taught to believe. We know now that the atom consists of a nucleus with a positive charge, electrons with a negative charge, and a large proportion of empty space. Nobody knows of what this empty space consists, but many of the foremost thinkers of this age, such as Sir James Jeans, Einstein, and Sir Oliver Lodge, have more than hinted that this empty space is filled with 'the stuff of consciousness', the guiding principle or the life-force which is believed to interpenetrate all matter. It is a sobering thought that where there apparently exists an intelligent and conscious life-force, this force must find its source in an intelligent and conscious Being. This can be none other than the life of the Creator itself, which alone provides life to all creation, as mentioned in John 1:4 'In Him was life; . . . '

Science, therefore, may not only be *affirming* religion, but may also be delivering the coup de grâce to the materialistic philosophy. It would appear that medical scientists in America, at the San Francisco General Hospital, have been doing exactly that; they have produced 'scientific evidence' that prayer works, and that prayer does something to make people healthier! These facts are revealed in a book by Larry Dorsey[14], an American doctor who describes himself as 'a typical product of the American Medical School'. He was, however, so deeply shaken with the results and implications of the findings at the San Francisco General Hospital that he now writes and lectures about them full-time.

Dr Hay would have welcomed these findings; he was very much aware of the need for the harmony of the whole man when he wrote: '. . . do not forget that the spiritual man is the first man, the mental man the second, and the physical the third man, and only when these second and third are in harmony can there be a proper spiritual state.'

There are signs and portents today in many directions of new vision and dedication among individuals and their societies, especially of a growing and salutary awareness *as never before* of the vital importance to health and happiness of right eating and right thinking.

It would appear from these signs and portents that the 'new health era' so dear to Dr Hay's heart has well and truly begun.

What Some Doctors Say

More than 200 years ago Voltaire wrote: 'We put medicines about which we know little, into bodies about which we know less, to cure diseases about which we know nothing at all.'

Sadly, many modern medicines are not doing the good that was expected of them but doing harm that was not expected of them. Moreover, despite the many magnificent triumphs of medical practice today, the main killing and crippling degenerative diseases are remaining stubbornly resistant to modern therapies.

It is, therefore, heartening to know that the nutritional research of many medical pioneers during the past six or seven decades, the recent enormous advances in understanding of cell and molecular biology, and the new biochemical methods of estimating vitamin deficiencies, have established beyond doubt the vital importance of adequate, sound nutrition to health and to the *prevention* of disease.

Regrettably, there is still a serious reluctance by conventional medicine to recognize the crucial role of diet, and this is still disregarded. One very plausible reason for this has been put forward by a noted

American doctor friend, Miles H. Robinson: 'It is too humiliating to admit that many of the diseases which are being treated so profitably and inadequately by orthodox methods might be helped, cured, or actually prevented by adequate nutrition.'

Nevertheless, it is encouraging to find that more and more members of the medical profession are proving for themselves the vital role of 'adequate' nutrition, and many are advocating the principles of wholefood nutrition at home – if not always for their patients.

It is even more encouraging to find that one-time medical sceptics of the Hay System are now advocating it to their patients, and an increasing number are personally putting it into practice. I was, therefore, delighted and honoured when Dr Kenneth Vickery kindly offered to write a contribution for a final chapter in which a few 'medical converts' could have their say about food combining.

I feel particularly honoured that this offer came from Dr Vickery – no one is more eminently qualified to write about health issues. Lately Medical Officer of Health and Director of Public Health of a health resort, National Chairman of the Royal Institute of Public Health and now Vice-President, he has spent a lifetime crusading for better health care, particularly in relation to our eating habits and properly grown 'real' food as opposed to food polluted with suspect additives and deficient in vital health-promoting nutrients – 'deplete food' as he termed it. His work over some 45 years has placed him way ahead of his time in community medicine.

I would like, here, to express my gratitude and

thanks to Dr Vickery, and to the other contributors –
Walter W. Yellowlees, J. Michael Midgley, Hans C.
Moolenburgh, Jan de Vries and Ronald Livingston
– for their valuable contributions to this chapter.

Dr Kenneth Vickery (OStJ, MD, FFCM, DPH) Hon. Consultant in Public Health

For some 60 years or more Doris Grant has been
a consistent and effective influence in the better-
ment of the integrity of our daily food.

In addition to newspaper and magazine articles, her message has been carried in a series of
bestselling books; like *Your Daily Bread*, 1944,
which is as valid today as the day it was written.

The main thrust of all her first 10 or more
books was the vital importance to health of the
wholeness, freshness, minimal processing and
organic nurture of the familiar components of
everyday eating. Each of these books, I now realize, mentioned her view that it was desirable to
be selective, regarding the items of food which
were taken together at any given meal. Desirous
as I was in public health education to achieve the
adoption of whole and unsophisticated food, I
confess that I paid little attention to the question of their combination in the diet. Indeed,
round about 1984, when she came out with
Food Combining for Health (with Jean Joice), my
scepticism surfaced and I was worried that she
was going off course down a side alley. I may say
that some other doctors who valued her overall

contribution were of the same view. How could these alleged enormous benefits possibly stem from whether or not one ate bread, potatoes, butter, meat and vegetables and a sweet course at one and the same time? A bit of indigestion sometimes, may be, but that's about all!

'From 1984 on, Doris Grant – with the help of Jean Joice – was now concentrating her main educative effort on the same aspect of food and health about which she wrote so enthusiastically and regularly in a national Sunday newspaper in 1936 and 1937. This was the food combining thesis of an American physician, Dr Hay, who had arrived at this, but also the importance of wholefood, by personal experience arising from his former ill health.

'Doris Grant evidently received great feed-back from the public (about three to five hundred letters a week) over her pre-war articles which brought Dr Hay to London and induced her to write *The Hay System Menu Book* (1937) giving recipes and menus of the Hay diet appropriate to the British housewife.

'This was the beginning in the UK of good publicity for Dr Hay (whose life was sadly curtailed by an accident) but nothing like the impact now reached with the publication of five editions of *Food Combining for Health* and 80 reprints, over half a million copies sold, and some 140 appearances in *The Sunday Times* lists of bestsellers.

'This record alone has been enough to make erstwhile scoffers like me think again. What really tops it all is the enormous unsolicited feedback, which the authors have received, of case histories of improved health (running into thousands of letters over the years). This has also impressed other sceptical doctors. We may not fully understand how it works, but clearly the proof of the pudding is in the eating thereof . . . .

'It has been truly said that whilst honour is due to the originator of a winning concept scarcely less honour is due to the disciple who grasps the idea and makes it available and understandable to the needful public. All honour to the success story of the Hay/Grant diet.

'It is probable that *Food Combining for Health* has been more influential in changing for the good the lifestyle of more people than any other "health" book in the twentieth century.

'Perhaps one of the most exciting potentials of giving the body a better chance to digest and metabolize the many components of food now so freely available, is the experience of many of an undoubted improvement in the precious immune system.

'At a time when low grade and endemic organisms are more and more involved in clinical illness, there is at long last a dawning realization in orthodox medicine that what really matters is not the germs which are ubiquitous and always with us, but the sustained power to resist their onslaught – the integrity of immune systems.

'Health professionals, and doctors in particular, are indeed liable to be very sceptical about "new" ideas relating to health and disease. This is understandable, given the constant stream of "new" cures, "new" treatments and especially "new" diets foisted on an all-too-gullible public. So many people are beset by problems which are resistant to orthodox medicine that they are ever-ready to clutch at straws.

'To hedge against being carried away by "nine day wonders", some of which may be positively harmful, the medical profession clings to the scientific method and the discipline of the double-blind trial. Not until a new thesis has been tried and tested, and tested again, by lengthy, demanding and time-consuming procedures, can there be any change in medical direction, and then only tentatively, in case it comes to nothing in the long term.

'Sadly, this kind of testing is most difficult, if not impossible, to apply to the one subject which has the potential for the greatest influence for good or ill on human health, i.e. that of the food we eat. Notwithstanding the personal experience of many, and of related epidemiological findings of races and nations, the health professions remain inhibited to countenance change in the absence of scientific experiments which may be impracticable – and it is not as if the status quo, in this case the nation's appalling diet, was arrived at in the first place by scientific method.

'A classic case is the observation of Dr Thomas Allinson, well over 100 years ago, that the poverty of nutrients in the bread and flour of the people of the East End of London was a major cause of their manifest ill health. He devoted his life to encouraging people towards simple wholegrain foods, and persuaded bakers to provide inexpensive wholewheat loaves. He was dubbed a crank and a charlatan, and was struck off the medical register for his pains!

'His torch was carried into the twentieth century by a few courageous pioneers against scepticism, ridicule, vested interest and indifference. White bread, a convenient product of the steel roller mills, continued to be publicized as the bread the people want and like and is "good for you". As recently as 1933, an eminent surgeon, Sir William Arbuthnot Lane, also lost his place in the medical register by remaining determined to continue to educate the public in healthy eating.

'To this day, as we approach the twenty-first century – and in spite (at long last) of the Department of Health's encouragement towards less refined cereals – it is sadly the case that white bread, white flour and sugary comestibles remain the norm for millions who desperately need the refined-out fibre, vitamins, minerals and proteins of wholegrain products.

'Experimental evidence of better health of races, sects, individuals, and in institutions where wholefood is the norm, has been there to be heeded over the whole of the century, but it has been blindly ignored, and continues to be so. As recently as 1970 a much quoted Professor of Nutrition was still advising *Times* readers that the issue of brown versus white bread was no more than colour prejudice!

'My fervent wish is that Doris Grant's *Food Combining for Life: The Health Success of the Century* is not only celebrated in its own right, as well as honouring her at the time of a landmark birthday, but also that the health professions grasp that, so far as the food habits of the nation are concerned, there are more effective ways (like massive personal experience) of arriving at necessary change than waiting for the results of double-blind feeding trials which may be impossible to devise.'

Dr Walter W. Yellowlees
(MC, MB, Ch.B, FRCGP)

'Digestive complaints bring thousands of unhappy patients daily to their GPs. For some, a precise diagnosis – peptic ulcer, hiatus hernia, "irritable bowel syndrome", and so on – will be possible. But for many, no explanation for their misery will be found; they will be given a variety of pills and potions and encouraged to soldier on.

'The same goes for those suffering from "rheumatic complaints"; in only a minority of cases will the GP be able to give a precise diagnosis. As neither the common digestive nor rheumatic disorders are life threatening, their nationwide numbers are not precisely known, but probably they account for about a quarter of all cases arriving at the door of our GPs.

'Mrs Grant is convinced that the lives of people in the grip of "rheumatism" or "indigestion" and other common complaints associated with food intolerance can be transformed by the simple dietary changes advised in the Food Combining way of eating. This applies whether or not a precise diagnosis has been made.

'The "simple dietary changes" come under two headings; the first follows the teaching of McCarrison and Cleave – fresh whole food instead of the refined, highly processed products beloved of modern consumers. The second requires changes in the way foods are combined at mealtimes.

'The success of Food Combining, detailed in this book, calls urgently for careful research. That Dr Hay's theory of human digestion, on which Food Combining is based, does not fully accord with present-day teaching, seems to me to make the call for research all the more urgent. If the healing power of Food Combining was confirmed and achieved wide acceptance in the NHS, the relief of suffering and saving of wealth would be incalculable.'

Dr J. Michael Midgley
(MB, Ch.B, MRCGP, MBKSTS)

'Nearly 30 years ago, whilst running a single-handed general practice, I developed ME (Myalgic encephalomyelitis) after a flu injection. This resulted in persistent extreme weariness, insomnia, numerous allergies to food additives, grasses, trees and pollens, and a Candida albicans infection of the gut. Such conditions are common complications of ME.

'Over the years I tried many different treatments, some of which enabled me to take slow steps towards recovery. One of these treatments was the Hay Diet. This produced an immediate and marked step forward, improving both my energy levels and my sleep.

'The Hay Diet is a very easy and wholesome diet to follow. You need only to give up peanuts, pulses and refined sugar! It's all in the combining of foods. I would certainly recommend it to anyone with a long standing illness, subject to their own GP's approval of course. It can do no harm and may well do a lot of good.'

Dr H.C. Moolenburgh (ARTS)

'Many times during the week patients ask me about their digestive troubles – one of the plagues of our time. A special group are those with hypoglycaemia, with their anxieties, dizzy spells, sudden headaches, etc. In most cases I do not order any remedies. I ponderously put Doris Grant's book *Food Combining for Health* before their astonished faces and say: "Buy this," (happily there exists a Dutch translation), "read it and do it."

'And often, as soon as two months later, grateful patients tell me that their complaints for the first time in years are either gone or else greatly diminished. Some say rather angrily: "Why did no one ever mention this way of life to me before?"

'Happily my partner in practice is a fervent fan of the food combining principle, so my patients – when coming to her with a book prescription – receive an enthusiastic briefing. I should not like to do without food combining in general practice.'

Jan de Vries (DHoMed, DOMRO, NDMRN, DAc, MBAcA)

'During my 35 years of practice, I often heard about food combining and, in particular, the subject was often raised at the numerous lectures I gave. Subsequently, I read several books about it and spoke to several people about it. However, it was only when I discovered Doris's absolutely wonderful book *Food Combining for Health*, co-authored with Jean Joice, that I was able to impart further knowledge on the subject to my patients and audiences. Not only was the book intelligently written but it was also translated into seven other languages. My respect and admiration for Doris was further strength-ened when I later had the privilege of some correspondence with her.

'When I wrote my book *Stomach and Bowel Disorders*, which has a foreword by Hayley Mills, I had the privilege of meeting Sir John Mills a few times. He spoke very highly of the Hay System of food combining, as he had incorporated it into his very busy and exciting life, and he reported the tremendous benefits that had occurred as a result of this. When patients are willing to follow the advice, it is amazing to see what can be achieved.

'I have written with the greatest pleasure to Doris Grant a few times, stating my admiration for how much she has done to help human suffering. Let's be honest, as Hippocrates so well said, "Your food must be your medicine and your medicine, your food". This is indeed where it all started, and if we look after our body chemistry well, with the right foods and the correct combination of foods, we will undoubtedly have a good energy output.

'The Hay Diet is not mathematics, it is just common sense, and there is nothing common about common sense, so I very happily recommend the Hay principles. I especially recommend the advice to just try it, as I know from past experience that it will be successful.

Dr Ronald Livingston (MB, BS, MFHom)

'What can I add to these glowing testimonials that has not been expressed by my distinguished colleagues? On a personal note I can add that I have been privileged to know Doris Grant – a wonderful lady – for nearly 40 years.

'I first heard about the Hay Diet when my medical Uncle Sam announced that he was "consuming" it, and I could not understand as a little boy why such a well built man was eating hay!

'I and my family, and as many of my patients

as I can persuade, are living examples of the tremendous value of this nutritional regime.'

How this chapter – and indeed the whole book – would have delighted Dr Hay!

References

Chapter 2

1. Yellowlees, W. W. *A Doctor in the Wilderness*, Janus Publishing Ltd, 1993
2. Bryce-Smith, Derek, and Hodgkinson, Liz *The Zinc Solution*, Century Acorn
3. McDowal, R. G. S. *Handbook of Physiology and Biochemistry* (42nd edn), John Murray, London
4. Munro, Daniel *Man Alive You're Half Dead!*, Bartholomew House Inc., 1950
5. Pavlov, Ivan *The Work of the Digestive Glands*, Charles Griffen & Company Limited, 1910
6. Rodale, J. I. *Natural Health, Sugar and the Criminal Mind*, Pyramid Books, New York
7. Collings, Jillie *Life Forces*, New English Library, 1991
8. Stewart, G. T. 'Dogma Disputed, Limitations of the Germ Theory', *Lancet*, 18 May 1968
9. *Sunday Times* article by Neville Hodgkinson, 31 January 1993
10. Luria, Dr 'The T2 Mystery', *Sc Amer*, vol. 192 (April 1955), pp. 92–98

11. Voisin, Andre *Soil, Grass and Cancer*, Crosby, Lockwood & Son Limited, 1959

12. Yamafugi, K. and Shirozu, Y. *Biochemische Z.*, vol. 317 (1944), p. 94; Yamafugi, K. and Fujiki, T.*Biochemische Z.*, vol. 318 (1944), pp. 101–106

13. Howard, Albert *Farming and Gardening for Health or Disease*, Faber & Faber, 1945

14. Biskind, Morton S. 'On Certain Aspects of the Origins and Treatments of Communicable Disease, with Particular Reference to Viruses', 1955

15. World Health Organisation *Diet, Nutrition and the Prevention of Chronic Diseases*, WHO Technical Series No. 797

16. Gibson, Sheila 'Effects of Fluoride on Immune System Function', *Complementary Medical Research*,vol. 6 (1992), pp. 111–113

17. Schauss, Alex *Diet, Crime and Delinquency*, Parker House Co., 1980

18. Schacter, Stanley *The Stop Smoking Diet* by J. Ogle, London, Sphere, 1984

19. Holford, Patrick *Green Cuisine*, February/March 1989

20. Wright, Celia *The Wright Diet*, Grafton Books, 1989

Chapter 4

1. Douglas, N. and Heathcote, A. *The Book of Earthly Delights* Compendium Pty Ltd, Australia, 1976

2. Cleave, T. L. *The Saccharine Disease*, Bristol, John Wright & Sons Ltd, 1974

3. Pavlov, Ivan *The Work of the Digestive Glands*, Charles Griffen & Co. Ltd, 1910

4. Picton, Lionel James *Liverpool Medico-Chirurgical Journal* (1931)
5. Collings, Jillie *The Ordinary Person's Guide to EXTRAORDINARY HEALTH*, Aurum Press Ltd, 1993
6. Van Straten, Michael and Griggs, Barbara *The Superfoods Diet Book*, Dorling Kindersley, 1992

Chapter 6

1. Trine, Ralph W. *In Tune with the Infinite*, Keats Publishing Inc., 1973
2. Jafolla, Richard and Mary *Nourishing the Life Force* Unity Books, Unity Village, Missouri. (Obtainable in the UK from Unity, 11 Boyn Hill Avenue, Maidenhead, Berks, SL6 4ET)
3. McCarrison, Robert 'Cantor Lectures', delivered before the Royal Society of Arts, 1936 – published as *Nutrition and Health*, McCarrison Society, 1982
4. Sinclair, Hugh 'World Health Day Speech', *British Medical Journal*, 14 December 1957
5. Cannon, Geoffrey and Walker, Caroline *The Observer*, 27 January and 3 February 1985
6. Taylor, Brent *The Lancet*, December 1984
7. Butler, Dr 'Nutrition and the Prevention of Physical Degeneration', McCarrison Society 14th Annual Conference, 1984
8. *Fit for Life*, Command 6684, HMSO
9. *The Health of the Nation*, Registrar General's Statistical Review 1931, and OPCS 1991
10. Westlake, Aubrey *Life Threatened*, London, Vincent Stuart, 1967

11. Price, Weston A. *Nutrition and Physical Degeneration*, The Academy of Applied Nutrition, Los Angeles, California, 1945

12. Mansfield, Dr Peter and Munro, Dr Jean *Chemical Children*, Century, 1987

13. Mackarness, Richard *Not All In the Mind*, Pan Books Ltd, 1976

14. Dorsey, Larry *Healing Words*, HarperCollins, 1993

Recommended Reading

Titles followed by an asterisk (•) contain information about, and/or recipes for, food combining.

Bartram, Thomas *Nature's Plan for Your Health*, Blandford Press, 1984

Bryce-Smith, Derek and Hodgkinson, Liz *The Zinc Solution*, Century-Arrow, 1986

Cilento, Lady Phyllis, MB, BS *You Don't Have to be Sick*, Keats Publishing Inc., 1984

Cleave, T. L. *The Saccharine Disease*, John Wright & Sons Ltd, Bristol, 1974

Collings, Jillie *Life Forces: Guidelines for a Healthy Life on a Polluted Planet*, New English Library, 1991*

Collings, Jillie *The Ordinary Person's Guide to Extraordinary Health*, New English Library, 1993*

de Vries, Jan *Nature's Gift of Food*, Mainstream Publishing Co. Ltd

de Vries, Jan *Viruses, Allergies and the Immune System*, Mainstream Publishing Co. Ltd, 1988

Dorsey, Larry *Healing Words*, HarperCollins, 1993

Elliot, Rose *Vegetarian Slimming*, The Vegetarian

Slimming Plan for Food Combining, Chapmans, 1991[*]

Feingold, Ben F. *Why Your Child is Hyperactive*, Random House, NY, 1993

Goodman, Sandra *Vitamin C – The Master Nutrient*, Keats Publishing Inc., USA (UK Distributors: Ashgrove Press, Bristol)

Graham, Judy *Evening Primrose Oil*, Thorsons, 1984

Grant, Doris and Joice, Jean *Food Combining for Health*, Thorsons, 1984

Griggs, Barbara *Zest for Life*, Ebury Press, 1989[*]

Hanssen, Maurice *E for Additives*, Thorsons, 1988

Hay, William Howard *A New Health Era*, Harrap (out of print, but second-hand copies may be obtainable from second-hand bookshops)

Health: State-of-the-Art (An important new quarterly 'designed to help health professionals stay informed about the burgeoning fields spanning the disciplines of complementary medicine.' From: Health Research, 6 Alfred Road, Windmill Hill, Bristol B63 4LE. Tel: 0117 9635109. Fax: 0117 9538069)[*]

Hodgson, Joan *A Book of Health and Healing*, White Eagle Publishing Trust, 1983[†]

Jafolla, Richard and Mary-Alice *Nourishing the Life Force*, Unity Books, Unity Village, Missouri, 1985. (A magnificent way of working with life forces, treating body, mind and spirit.)

Joice, Jean and Le Tissier, Jackie *The Food Combining*

[†] Just before *Food Combining for Life* went to press, *Health: State of-the-Art* was incorporated with *Positive Health* and is now published under that name.

for Health Cookbook, Thorsons, 1994

Kenton, Leslie *The Biogenic Diet*, Century Press, 1986*

Lacy, Prof. Richard *Unfit for Human Consumption*, Souvenir Press Ltd, 1991

Le Tissier, Jackie *Food Combining for Vegetarians*, Thorsons, 1992

Lidolt, Erwina *The Food Combining Cookbook*, Thorsons, 1989

Mabey, David, Gear, Alan and Jackie (eds) *Thorsons Organic Consumer Guide*, Thorsons, 1990

Mackarness, Dr Richard *Chemical Victims*, Pan Books Ltd, 1980

Mansfield, Dr Peter and Munro, Dr Jean *Chemical Children*, Century Press, 1987

Marsden, Kathryn *The Food Combining Diet*, Thorsons, 1993

Marshall, Janette *The Ultimate ACE Diet*, Vermillion, 1994

McCarrison, Sir Robert and Sinclair, H. M. *Nutrition and Health*, McCarrison Society, 1982

McEoin, Beth *Healthy by Nature*, Thorsons, 1994

Meek, Jennifer *Immune Power*, Optima, 1980

Montignac, Michel *Montignac Recipes and Menus*, Artulen UK, 1994*

Moolenburgh, Hans *Fluoride The Freedom Fight*, Mainstream Publishing Co. Ltd, 1987

Newbound, Maurice *Catering for Health and Special Diets*, G. S. Publications, Chardstock House, Chard, Somerset TA20 2TL*

Pauling, Linus *How to Live Longer and Feel Better*, W. H. Freeman & Co., 1986

Picton, Dr Lionel James OBE *Thoughts on Feeding*, Faber & Faber, 1946

Polunin, Miriam *The New Cookbook*, Macdonald, 1984

Positive Health (A new-style bi-monthly health magazine published by Positive Health, 6 Alfred Road, Windmill Hill, Bristol, B63 4LE. Tel: 0117 9635109. Fax: 0117 9538069)

Shreeve, Caroline M. *Fish Oil the Life Saver*, Thorsons, 1992

Spong, Tim and Peterson, Vicki *Food Combining*, Prism Press, 1993

Stone, Dr Irwin *The Healing Factor: Vitamin C Against Disease*, Grosset & Dunlap

Van Straten, Michael and Griggs, Barbara *The Superfoods Diet Book*, Dorling Kindersley, 1992*

Webb, Tony and Lang, Dr Tim *Food Irradiation: The Facts*, Thorsons, 1987

Wright, Celia *The Wright Diet*, Grafton Books, 1989*

Yellowlees, Dr W. W. *A Doctor in the Wilderness*, Janus Publishing Ltd, 1993*

Yudkin, John *Pure, White and Deadly: The Problem of Sugar*, Penguin, 1988

Useful Addresses

Vitamins C and E in powder form:
Vitamin E and Evening Primrose Oil In capsules:
  Renahall Ltd, 61 Lime Tree Avenue, Rugby,
  CV22 7QT
  Tel: 01788 11454 (Mail order service)

Chicory
  Northumbrian Fine Foods Plc, Dukesway,
  Team Valley, Tyneside NE11 0QP
  Tel: 0191 4870070
  (Stocked by most health food shops.)

Pesticide-free organic chocolate
  (for the occasional treat!)
  Green & Black's Dark Chocolate.
  Stockists include: Holland and Barrett; Safeway;
  Sainsburys.

Organic Honey
  Pure Honey Supplies Co., Mildon House,
  Cedar Avenue, Enfield, Middlesex

Organic Food Services, Ash, Churston Ferrers, Brixham, S. Devon

Organic raisins and sultanas, organic rice, porridge oats and tea
Healthy Fayre, 2 Newbury Court, Gillingham, Dorset
Tel: 01747 825683

Organic Bran
Nicholas Terrence, The Water Mill, Little Salkeld, Penrith, Cumbria
Tel: Langworthy 523

Organic wholefoods – everything organic
Dried and fresh fruits, vegetables, saladings, meat and poultry.
Wholefoods Ltd, 24 Paddington Street, London W1M 4DR
Tel: 0171 935 3924

Organic yogurt
Rachel's Yogurt, Safeway, Gateway/Somerfield and Sainsburys.
Rachel's Dairy Ltd
Tel: 01970 625805

Organic Flour
Dove's Farm Foods Ltd (Mail order service)
Salisbury Rd., Hungerford, Berkshire RG17 0RF
Tel: 01488 684880

Food combining food chart
A coloured and decorative food chart, identical to that in

Food Combining for Health, *is available for day-to-day use and is particularly helpful to beginners in planning Hay System meals. It costs £2 (plus postage) and can be obtained from*

   Nora Wingate, Gorse Cottage, Furze Hill,
   Nr. Fordingbridge, Hants, SP6 2PU
   Tel: 01425 657813

The Hyperactive Society Children's Support Group for Hyperactivity, Allergies and Learning Difficulties.
   Tel: 01903 725182

Index